"It's time to open the therapy room door, step outside, and use the great outdoors to help those who seek our counsel. This comprehensive text, written by experts around the world, shows you how."
—*Scott Miller, PhD, founder of the*
International Center for Clinical Excellence and
coauthor of Better Results: Using Deliberate
Practice to Improve your Therapeutic Effectiveness

"In public health, the importance of human interactions with outdoor and nature-based settings is emerging as critically important to physical and mental well-being. Although focused on therapy, this book's application and utility for health promotion practitioners and researchers is evident. I will absolutely be recommending this text to my students and colleagues involved in outdoor and nature-based interventions."
—*Patti-Jean Naylor, PhD, professor in the School of*
Exercise Science, Physical and Health Education
at the University of Victoria, and international expert
on children's physical activity, healthy eating,
and applying implementation science

"Outdoor therapies are fast evolving. We gradually realize that we do not have to confine ourselves to the therapy room; the outside world offers beautiful therapy opportunities. If you are interested in this growing field, this book will provide you with a great variety of topics and insights to enrich your thoughts and work."
—*Itai Ivtzan, PhD, associate professor at*
Naropa University and author of
Awareness is Freedom: The Adventure
of Psychology and Spirituality

"This book recognizes the relationship between humans and nature as fundamental to human experience, and perhaps most important for the practitioner and policy maker alike, this book brings together the many streams of nature-based interventions and shows how underneath the superficial appearance is a fundamental reality that is vital for the future of the planet. This integrated approach is needed to support the field and inform all stakeholders of the possibilities inherent within outdoor therapies."
—*Eric Brymer, PhD, associate professor and*
author of One Health: The Well-being
Impacts of Human-Nature Relationships

T0386478

Outdoor Therapies

Drawing on the leading voices of international researchers and practitioners, *Outdoor Therapies* provides readers with an overview of practices for the helping professions.

Sharing outdoor approaches ranging from garden therapy to wilderness therapy and from equine-assisted therapy to surf therapy, Harper and Dobud have drawn common threads from therapeutic practices that integrate connection with nature and experiential activity to redefine the "person-in-environment" approach to human health and well-being. Readers will learn about the benefits and advantages of helping clients get the treatment, service, and care they need outside of conventional, office-based therapies.

Providing readers with a range of approaches that can be utilized across a variety of practice settings and populations, this book is essential reading for students, practitioners, theorists, and researchers in counseling, social work, youth work, occupational therapy, and psychology.

Nevin J. Harper, PhD, has been involved in adventure education and outdoor therapy practices for more than 25 years. His research and practice focuses on active, embodied, and ecological approaches for therapy, health, and well-being.

Will W. Dobud, PhD, MSW, is a social work lecturer at Charles Sturt University and has been involved in outdoor therapy in the United States, Australia, and Norway. His research is focused on participant experiences in care and improving outcomes in the outdoor therapies.

Outdoor Therapies

An Introduction to Practices, Possibilities, and Critical Perspectives

Edited by Nevin J. Harper
and Will W. Dobud

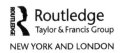

Routledge
Taylor & Francis Group

NEW YORK AND LONDON

First published 2021
by Routledge
52 Vanderbilt Avenue, New York, NY 10017

and by Routledge
2 Park Square, Milton Park, Abingdon, Oxon, OX14 4RN

Routledge is an imprint of the Taylor & Francis Group, an informa business

Library of Congress Cataloging-in-Publication Data
Names: Harper, Nevin J., editor. | Dobud, Will W., editor.
Title: Outdoor therapies: introduction to practices, possibilities, and critical perspectives / edited by Nevin J. Harper and Will W. Dobud.
Description: New York, NY: Routledge, 2021. | Includes bibliographical references and index. Identifiers:
LCCN 2020017667 | ISBN 9780367365714 (hardback) |
ISBN 9780367365707 (paperback) | ISBN 9780429352027 (ebook)
Subjects: LCSH: Adventure therapy. | Nature—Therapeutic use. | Ecopsychiatry.
Classification: LCC RC489.A38 O98 2021 |
DDC 616.89/165—dc23
LC record available at https://lccn.loc.gov/2020017667

ISBN: 978-0-367-36571-4 (hbk)
ISBN: 978-0-367-36570-7 (pbk)
ISBN: 978-0-429-35202-7 (ebk)

Typeset in Sabon
by codeMantra

Contents

Acknowledgments

First, we would like to thank the international collection of scholars who contributed their time and energy to this introductory text. This collection of chapters, penned by notable authors from Canada, Australia, Belgium, USA, Norway, and South Korea, spans the diverse and exciting range of outdoor therapies. We also give thanks to our colleagues, clients, and the field's thought leaders and practitioners who have informed and guided our work over the years. Last, to our families for their love, support, and sharing our life's adventures together.

About the Contributors

Scott Bandoroff, PhD, is a psychologist specializing in the use of adventure therapy for the treatment of teens and families. In addition to his work as a clinician, he has served as a clinical supervisor, internship director, consultant, and trainer. Scott leads wilderness family intensives and pioneered the Clinical First Responder Training to advance the clinical skills of direct care staff working in therapeutic outdoor settings.

Cathryn Carpenter, PhD, is currently working as a curriculum development specialist at Deakin University, Melbourne, Australia. She has worked within the outdoor education and adventure therapy profession with a focus on health and well-being for more than 40 years. She has lectured at universities, been a ski instructor and adventure guide, is a past president of the Victoria Outdoor Education Association, and was long-involved in the leadership of the Adventure Therapy International Committee.

Daniel L. Cavanaugh, LCSW, is a licensed clinical social worker in Portland, USA and a PhD candidate at Michigan State University's School of Social Work. Daniel has integrated adventure therapy techniques into school and community-based mental health practice with youth and families. Daniel also teaches social work students how to use experiential interventions in their clinical practice.

Nicholas XEMŦOLTW̱ Claxton, PhD, was born and raised in Saanich (W̱SÁNEĆ) Territory. He has a master's degree in Indigenous Governance and a PhD in Education from the University of Victoria, Canada. Nicholas is an assistant professor in the School of Child and Youth Care at the University of Victoria and Chief of the Tsawout Nation. His research interests are in revitalizing traditional environmental knowledge and land-based practices of Indigenous peoples.

Megan E. Delaney, PhD, LPC, is an assistant professor in the department of Professional Counseling at Monmouth University where she created and teaches courses for the Ecotherapy certificate. Therapy Without Walls, LLC is her private practice. Her research explores the influence of the natural world on our mental health and the use of Ecotherapy. Megan's book, *Nature is nurture: Counseling and the natural world*, is published via Oxford University Press.

Will W. Dobud, MSW, PhD, is a lecturer with Charles Sturt University and the founder and director of the adventure therapy program, True North Expeditions, in Australia. Will is a representative of the Australian Association for Bush Adventure Therapy and has been involved in adventure therapy programming internationally since 2005.

Thomas J. Doherty, PsyD, is a clinical and environmental psychologist based in Portland, USA. He has written numerous publications on nature-based therapies, the restorative effects of outdoor experiences, and the mental health impacts of climate change. He is a fellow of the American Psychological Association, a past president of the Society for Environmental, Population, and Conservation Psychology, and founding editor of the journal *Ecopsychology*. He also founded, directed, and taught in the Ecopsychology Certificate program at Lewis & Clark Graduate School.

Carina Ribe Fernee, PhD, is a researcher and practitioner at Sørlandet Hospital in Norway. She has been involved in the implementation of outdoor therapy in adolescent mental health care since 2013. Carina is a representative of the Nordic Outdoor Therapy Network and co-chair of the Adventure Therapy International Committee.

Leiv Einar Gabrielsen, PhD, is a researcher and practitioner at Sørlandet Hospital in Norway. He has been involved in the implementation of outdoor therapy in adolescent mental health care since 2012. Leiv is a representative of the Nordic Outdoor Therapy Network, an honorary member of the Adventure Therapy International Committee, and the managing director of Nordic Dawn Adventures and Counselling, an outdoor therapy company.

Rebecca L. Haller, MS (HTM), is the director and lead instructor of the Horticultural Therapy Institute where she teaches horticultural therapy classes in affiliation with Colorado State University. She has developed and conducted vocational and therapeutic programs, written textbooks on the profession, and served as president and board member of the American Horticultural Therapy Association.

Nevin J. Harper, PhD, is an associate professor in the School of Child and Youth Care at the University of Victoria. His research, consulting, and training are in the areas of outdoor therapies, human-nature relationships, leadership, and risk management. Nevin is the founder of the Canadian Adventure Therapy Symposium and co-author of *Nature-based therapy: A practitioner's guide to working outdoors with children, youth and families* from New Society Publishers.

Juyoung Lee, PhD, is a professor of Landscape Architecture in Hankyong National University, South Korea. He is interested in the *interdisciplinary* research on the verification of health-related benefits of natural resources including vegetation, urban greenspace, water, and landscapes using psychological and physiological tools. His research focuses on evidence-based urban planning and design and forest therapy to improve human health.

Kaya Lyons, BAppSc (OT), is an occupational therapist driven to unlocking every child's unique abilities and achieving success in life. Kaya is director of Active OT 4 Kids and Camp 'Reset.' She has extensive experience working with children and families presenting with trauma, emotional and behavioral disorders, and complex needs. She values the importance of play, attachment, and movement.

Denise Mitten, PhD, is internationally recognized for her innovative scholarship in outdoor and environmental pedagogy, ethics, and gender. She has advocated for and written about caring and compassionate leadership since 1985. She is a widely experienced adventure guide, professor at Prescott College, author of *Natural environments and human health*, and co-editor of *Experiential education theory and practice* and *The Palgrave MacMillan international handbook of women and outdoor learning*.

Christine Lynn Norton, PhD, LCSW, is an associate professor of Social Work at Texas State University. She also serves as a research scientist with the Outdoor Behavioral Healthcare Center, examining wilderness and adventure therapy programs and practices. Her PhD is in Social Work and she has an MA in Social Service Administration and an MS in Experiential Education. Christine has over 20 years of experience working with youth and young adults in therapeutic wilderness programs, juvenile justice, schools, mentoring, and campus support programs.

Luk Peeters, MEdSci, has been working experientially outdoors since 1985. He holds a master's degree in educational sciences and is a Gestalt and Person-Centred therapist with specializations in Existential and in Group Psychotherapy. He is a staff member in a Person-Centred Therapy and Group Therapy training program. He also coordinates and facilitates an Adventure Therapy specialization training program in Belgium in collaboration with Outward Bound where he has been a trainer for more than 30 years. He is also a partner in the international Via Experientia network.

Jess Ponting, PhD, caught his first wave around age eight and became instantly addicted to the feeling of well-being the experience provided. He holds the world's first master's and PhD degrees focusing on the impacts of surf tourism, founded the International Association for Surf Research, and the Center for Surf Research at San Diego State University of which he is the director. Jess is a longtime advocate of the benefits of surfing for those who participate and researches, writes, and presents internationally on surf therapy, surf parks, and surf tourism.

Anita Pryor, PhD, trained in outdoor education and family therapy and was a canoe, raft, and ski guide in Australia and Austria before managing a drug treatment adventure therapy service for young people. Anita has been an active contributor to national and international adventure therapy networks for two decades, and currently co-directs Adventure Works Australia Ltd., a not-for-profit provider of bush adventure therapy interventions, research, and practitioner training.

Martin Ringer, MEd, is a member of the International Society for the Psychoanalytic Study of Organizations and founded the psychodynamic consultants' group Dynamics@Work. He was convener of the 1st International Adventure Therapy Conference (IATC) in 1997 and co-convened the 8th IATC in 2018. Martin's work on adventure therapy, experiential learning, and social dynamics is widely published and includes the book *Group action: The dynamics of groups in therapeutic, educational, and corporate settings* from Jessica Kingsley Publishers.

Kathryn Rose, MA, RCC, has been discovering the joys of experiential and nature-based approaches to working with children, youth, and families in nature for over ten years. She completed a master's degree in Transpersonal Counselling Psychology, with a specialization in Wilderness Therapy, from Naropa University in Colorado. Katy co-founded and is clinical director of Human-Nature Counselling and Consulting in Victoria, Canada, and is registered with the BC Association of Clinical Counsellors.

David Segal, MA, RCC, has provided therapeutic nature-based counselling for children, youth, and families for over 15 years. He offers presentations and workshops and has been contributing to the emerging field of eco-therapy through his work as a clinical counsellor and publishing articles in ecopsychology and counselling journals. He holds a master's degree in Child and Youth Care from the University of Victoria and is registered with the BC Association of Clinical Counsellors. Dave is co-founder and executive director of Human-Nature Counselling and Consulting in Victoria, Canada.

Kay Scott, PhD, LCSW-R, CASAC, is the associate vice-president for Behavioral Health Services at St. John's Riverside Hospital in Yonkers, NY (USA). She has twenty years of experience delivering animal-assisted interventions as well as teaching and evaluating canine/human teams delivering services to a variety of populations, including survivors of crisis and disaster. Her area of expertise is the use of canine-assisted therapies to support trauma-informed care. Kay holds degrees from Columbia and Fordham Universities.

Won Sop Shin, PhD, is a professor of social forestry at Chungbuk National University. He is a former Minister of Korea Forest Service and has been involved in many forest therapy research projects, the development of protected forest areas in forest therapy centers nationally, and in leadership with the International Society of Nature and Forest Medicine.

Anita R. Tucker, PhD, is an associate professor of Social Work at the University of New Hampshire. She is the Co-Coordinator of UNH's Dual Master's Degree in Social Work and Kinesiology: Outdoor Education, which prepares graduate students for careers in adventure and wilderness therapy. In addition, she is the associate director of the Outdoor Behavioral Healthcare Center for Research where she is responsible for the promotion of research, accreditation, and risk management in adventure therapy programs.

Heather White, LMSW, has worked within the human-animal interactions field for over a decade, incorporating both canines and equines in experiential interactions with individuals and groups and emphasizes mutually beneficial interactions for all species involved. Heather is the owner of AIM HAI, LLC, an animal-assisted interactions consulting company.

Disclaimer for Practice

This book is not a substitution for professional training and qualifications. Therapeutic work carries with it significant professional obligations and responsibilities. Taking your practice outside further increases your liability and needs to be taken on with the knowledge and competencies required to do so meaningfully and ethically. While you may be inspired to try activities and approaches suggested in this book, you must also take responsibility for ensuring the health and safety of your clients, that professional codes and standards are not compromised, and that you meet regulatory bodies approval for your work. It is assumed you will utilize knowledge gained from this book relative to your type and level of training, the mandate of your organization or practice, and to complement the helping skills you have already developed. The publisher, editors, and chapter authors hold no responsibility for any consequences of action taken as a result of the information contained in this book.

Part I

Foundations

Chapter 1

An Introduction to Outdoor Therapies

Nevin J. Harper and Thomas J. Doherty

Introduction

The Institute for Outdoor Learning in the United Kingdom recently released a statement of good practice for outdoor mental health interventions (Richards, Hardie, & Anderson, 2019). This publication, endorsed by the British Society of Lifestyle Medicine, provides guidelines for the "combining of mental health and well-being interventions with outdoor learning" (p. 1). This effort by Richards and colleagues exemplifies the desire we see among our international colleagues for a stronger confluence between psychological services and practices in the realm of environmental education, outdoor adventure, and nature-based therapies. In assembling this book, we hope for a similar outcome. We present this collection of outdoor therapies to assist mental health practitioners worldwide to go outside, be present to the elements, see the beauty in the forests, walk on the beaches, and explore health and well-being among the varied landscapes and species of their home places.

There is potential for great depth in thinking about the philosophy, ethics, and practice of outdoor therapies as forms of *ecotherapy* and as applied forms of *environmental psychology* (see Doherty, 2016; Doherty & Chen, 2016). On the surface, outdoor therapies obviously have philosophical and stylistic differences from commonly practiced indoor approaches. Outdoor therapies also have a different *neuropsychology*; we know that being active in stimulus-rich natural environments affects our brains and bodies differently than a sedentary and office-bound experience does (Berman, Stier, & Akcelik, 2019).

For our survey, we were interested in established outdoor therapeutic approaches that share common practices such as place-based learning, embodied experiences, therapeutic adventure, and nature-based stress reduction. We were also interested in revealing mental health practices that include nature and the outdoors as an active ingredient of healing. We predict that readers who take in the scope of outdoor therapy activities in this text—with chapters on wilderness therapy, horticultural therapy, equine therapy, outdoor occupational therapy, surf therapy, etc.—will come away with a new vision for counseling and therapy practice in the 21st century. We hope practitioners will try these experiences for themselves and reflect on the opportunities afforded to those they serve.

A Note on Culture and Privilege

In our approach to outdoor therapy, we were attentive to issues of cultural competency, bias, and privilege. There are many cultural lenses through which to view nature and outdoor experiences. These range from utilitarian 'wise-use' viewpoints that assume human dominance and mastery over nature to more humanistic and holistic approaches that assume kinship and shared value between humans, nature, and other species. This dominance-kinship tension is as old as humankind, reflected in historic and modern Indigenous cultures, and ethical debates about sustainability in technologically developed societies.

Few people are taught the skills to reflect on their environmental identity and values. So, these beliefs often remain implicit—leading to well-meaning but unconscious biases and unexamined privilege. If one has grown up with a utilitarian mindset that sees nature as a distant or threatening force to master, it is very difficult to imagine a safe experience of kinship and interbeing with nature. Conversely, if someone has grown up with healthy access to green spaces and developmental experiences in nature, it is easy to take these gifts for granted.

Why Take Therapy Outdoors?

Clients do not always find alignment between their needs and what is offered in therapy. In the case of young people, for example, half of the attempts at therapy fail (Neumann et al., 2010). While we cannot explain this problem in its entirety and researchers have attempted to do so (Garcia & Weisz, 2002), we can say confidently that a range of effective alternatives are available. This book describes a number of outdoor approaches to counseling, therapy, healing, wellness, and health promotion that positively contribute to psychosocial well-being, and physical, cognitive, and emotional functioning (Mygind et al., 2019).

This book also explains how outdoor therapies can bring the benefits of being outdoors into the counseling and therapy process and illustrates these benefits by describing a variety of unique approaches. We reconceptualize therapy to suggest that we, as a species, are endowed with an innate longing to be connected to nature and are often, by design, healthier and happier when we have access to compatible natural settings. Active engagement of the body in natural environments can mediate the process of therapy and contribute to its health-promoting outcomes (Maller, Townsend, Pryor, Brown, & St. Leger, 2005). At base, we propose that the mindset for and setting of outdoor therapies comprise an ideal approach to health and well-being for many (Wilson, Ross, Lafferty, & Jones, 2009; Wolsko & Lindberg, 2013). This is a shift in practice for therapists that requires additional knowledge and a willingness to alter conventional practices (Jordan & Marshall, 2010).

One criticism of the growing 'nature immersion for health' literature is that many recommendations or studies do not specify what encompassed the specific 'nature' conditions and exposure (Barnes et al., 2019). In this regard, you will find references throughout the chapters signifying positive outcomes that are awaiting replication and further development to enable wider practice. This is a common challenge for research in outdoor therapies, as well as all psychological studies. The power of outdoor therapies is only being revealed by theorists and practitioner-researchers willing to tackle the issue (see Fernee, Gabrielsen, Andersen, & Mesel, 2017). A second related criticism of the research on the benefits of exposure to nature is that little is known about long-term outcomes (Norwood et al., 2019), although knowledge is building on this front as well (Annerstedt & Währborg, 2011).

Our intention in compiling the practices described in this book is to share with readers the significant potential of outdoor approaches to health, healing, and well-being. We hope to inspire professionals in human-service and educational fields to consider engaging in these practices. We refrain from universal claims—such as 'being outdoors is good for everyone' or 'nature is healing.' Nature is a place where one can get a painful sunburn, become lost and scared, or become an environmental refugee in the wake of climate disasters. We acknowledge the limitations, both real and perceived, to moving a counseling practice outdoors, and yet advocate and encourage consideration to try.

Outdoor Therapies in Our Current Societal Context

In traditional societies, healing and medicine is based on herbal, spiritual, and community-oriented activities; it is all encompassing, holistic, and integral (Moodley & West, 2005). Across the world, some groups still adhere to these perennial practices while others are rediscovering them. However, healing practices in most 'developed' societies have shifted away from the realm of 'shaman-herbal-natural' and toward a 'medical-clinical-pharmaceutical' model. This is touted as advancement yet can also be seen as a loss: Loss of knowledge, loss of meaningful practice, loss of ways of being, and loss of ability to deal with illness in a natural way. Parallel to these shifts in healing practice, we are witness to an unprecedented and rapid acceleration of information sharing and technological advancements in modern societies. Living in a world of technological artifice can leave people functionally disconnected from experiences in the natural world, inhibit their knowledge of ecology, and promote an attenuated or even unhealthy relationship with the environments that sustain us on this planet (Harper, Harper, & Snowden, 2017).

Human societies have never experienced such heightened access to global knowledge sharing and movement of resources through multinational capitalism. Yet, collectively, we are plagued by persistent and growing mental health crises, sedentary lifestyle diseases such as diabetes and obesity, and a displacement of peoples due to genocide, political collapse, environmental crisis, and the ongoing effects of colonization on Indigenous peoples (Silove, Ventevogel, & Rees, 2017). A half-century ago, futurist Alvin Toffler (1984) proposed a condition called 'future shock' to describe "the shattering stress and disorientation that we induce in individuals by subjecting them to too much change in too short a time ... Our technological powers increase, but the side effects and potential hazards also escalate" (p. 12). Currently, with the impacts of the global climate crisis added to rapid technological change and normative environmental estrangement, we are now concerned with issues such as 'nature-deficit disorder,' 'eco-anxiety,' and 'solastagia.' Whether we will be able to adapt rapidly enough is in question.

If we take a selected snapshot of our current state of health, we can see a troubling reality:

- More than 55% of the population of earth now lives in urban settings (United Nations, 2018); North Americans spend approximately 90% of their days indoors and 5% in their cars (Klepeis et al., 2001). This places significant demands on our directed attention and other cognitive resources to safely and effectively navigate urban spaces (Kaplan & Berman, 2010).
- Accelerated rates of child and adult screen time are correlated with decreases in physical activity (Duncan, Vandelanotte, Caperchione, Hanley, & Mummery, 2012).
- Mental health and sedentary lifestyle diseases are rising in North America in what is considered an epidemic, including one in five youth diagnosed with anxiety or depression, and many more undiagnosed due to sub-threshold symptoms (Merikangas et al., 2010; Poitras et al., 2016; Wilmot et al., 2012).
- Global populations and life expectancy continue to rise across industrialized countries (Kontis et al., 2017), yet these gains are tempered by inequality across race and gender, with some groups being left behind (Geronimus, Bound, Waidmann, Rodriguez, & Timpe, 2019).

- Climate crises impact mental health with increased incidence of despair, anxiety, and sense of loss world-wide (Doherty & Clayton, 2011; Fritze, Blashki, Burke, & Wiseman, 2008).

The social and physical 'built' environments we spend time in have also been identified as important to human health. We can see this in environmental scans where toxins and air quality are measured; standing desks are being installed in offices to improve the health of sedentary workers, and plants and soothing colors are used for interior decorating to increase focus and wellness. If all these are indicators suggest our innate desire for more natural living (Kellert & Wilson, 1995), we ask why then is it often difficult to propose moving counseling and psychotherapy outdoors? Being outdoors is a necessary and integral part of human health which has been ignored by mainstream mental health promotion and therapy for too long. A growing body of evidence now supports time and activity in nature as positive for population health and well-being (Burls, 2007; Mygind et al., 2019), and to ameliorate specific mental and social health issues (Kondo, South, & Branas, 2015; Shanahan et al., 2019).

Our text is founded on a clear cultural critique: We, in modern technological societies, have ignored the role of nature and natural living for humans for too long, and this may hold more answers for our health and well-being than we currently give credit. Nature is a multi-dimensional net which encompasses, contains, and feeds us all. The air we breathe, the water we drink, the proteins, minerals, carbohydrates, and vitamins we absorb from our food are essential to our health and existence. These factors, however, are often taken for granted.

Outdoor Therapies and First Nations Cultures

One narrative surfacing throughout this book is that outdoor therapies address the need for alternatives to modern, office-based mental health approaches. There is no contesting that our recent experiences of accelerated urbanization and technification have had significant negative impacts (Gabrielsen & Harper, 2018). Many authors in our text describe practices that replicate or evoke 'old ways' of being such as growing food or choosing to burden oneself by carrying a backpack on a multi-day overland hike. Thus, while we look forward toward improved services for those in need of therapy, we are also drawing on our collective ancestral ways of being.

Research with First Nations groups in Canada has found that community health is improved where traditional languages and cultural practices have been retained or resurrected (Chandler & Lalonde, 1998). The effects of colonization and the systematic divorcing of First Nations from land-based practice are being redressed through resurgence activities which include land-based pedagogies and reconnection projects (Wildcat, McDonald, Irlbacher-Fox, & Coulthard, 2014). In Chapter 5, Indigenous scholar Nicholas XEMŦOLTW̱ Claxton shares an Indigenous land-based approach and highlights the reality that to many First Nations, the relationship to the land (and water) is THE primary relationship culturally—and central to Indigenous cosmology, health, well-being, and resurgence within their communities (Robbins & Dewar, 2011; Smith, Tuck, & Yang, 2019). Claxton provides knowledge and encouragement for non-Indigenous practitioners of outdoor therapies, especially those working on traditional Indigenous lands, to stay present to and acknowledge the history, stories, and place-based lessons in their work.

When honoring the First Nations context, outdoor therapists discover what a culture honoring of land, place-based knowledge, and close relationship with nature looks like. As Euro-western 'settlers,' they may also sense their innate cosmological connections to nature—a transcendent ecological experience that was suppressed during the rise of Christianity and Western traditions of science that effectively erased common earth-based *pagan* rituals and practices, arguably one of the roots of today's environmental crises (White Jr., 1967). From this perspective, the destruction of Europe's *sacred groves* carried over to colonizing practices in the 'New World' where lands were considered empty of civilized people (Terra Nullius), resources were exploited, and possession of the land *taken*. Resources were extracted to benefit colonizers, and Indigenous peoples were stripped of their places and cultural identity, resulting in generations of social and psychological suffering (Lavallee & Poole, 2010). We need to recognize and work toward ally-ship in restoring land-based practices across cultures and nations. Along the way, we will be challenged to examine how we as outdoor therapy practitioners may be privileged by our social locations and access to beautiful outdoor places and experiences that may be limited or harmful to others (Twine & Gardener, 2013).

Common Factors of Outdoor Therapies

All of the outdoor therapies shared in this book have bodies of empirical and conceptual literature supporting them, in many cases clear definitions of practice, and in some cases (e.g., horticultural therapy and forest therapy) professional associations and certification schemes. We are aware this may come as news to therapists unfamiliar with outdoor therapies. Indeed, even the authors in this text, experts in their individual pursuits, are being educated about the depth of other outdoor therapy approaches. Taken collectively, there is no universally recognized definition for outdoor therapies. There are, however, several common factors shared in some form by these approaches.

Outdoor Therapies Are Place Based

The physical location where clients and therapists meet is primarily outdoors. Regardless of theoretical approach or end goal, our chapters describe practices that take place outside of built structures, or that move outside as conditions allow. This place orientation, outdoors versus in, can improve outcomes for clients. Current reviews of research have shown nature exposure to improve cognition and affect for individuals with depression (Berman et al., 2012), and to promote positive changes in attention, memory, and mood (Norwood et al., 2019). The number of publications supporting human engagement with nature for enhancement of health has accelerated in recent years (e.g., Mygind et al., 2019). Clinical studies have shown improved immune function and cancer-fighting abilities for individuals walking in old growth forests (Li, 2010), while health and fitness studies have shown increased benefits of exercise outdoors versus indoors (Pasanen, Tyrväinen, & Korpela, 2014). This is a snapshot of the diverse scholarly and research efforts that strengthen the argument for spending more time outdoors, and, of course, we can be criticized for borrowing these findings to benefit promoting outdoor therapies. As more systematic reviews of the literature surface and more specific outdoor therapy research are conducted, we can become more confident in our claims of the benefits of these approaches for therapy and for general population health (Annerstedt & Währborg, 2011).

It is important to note that, while the outdoor environment is a primary element of outdoor therapies, outdoor therapists also work on the *threshold* between built and outdoor spaces. As Jordan and Marshall (2010) note, for some clients, and for certain clinical issues or difficult conversations, containment provided by an office setting is indicated. Thus, outdoor therapists can (1) initiate movement toward outdoor therapy sessions with a client, (2) work both indoors and outdoors, or (3) be an indoor therapist who *brings nature in* through the use of natural objects, focus on human-nature connections, and assignments of nature-based activities. Working across this spectrum is part of the art and science of outdoor therapies. One has to only envision the dark clouds of an oncoming rainstorm to consider how a retreat to a covered structure easily becomes a question of comfort and client care.

Outdoor Therapies Feature Active Bodily Engagement

A second element present in outdoor therapies is active physical engagement with the natural environment. Outdoor activity can increase attention (Taylor & Kuo, 2009), reduce stress (Jiang, Chang, & Sullivan, 2014), and provide general benefits for mental health (Bélanger et al., 2019). Learning is actively supported by bodily involvement with the environment (Corazon, Schilhab, & Stigsdotter, 2011; Poitras et al., 2016), and it is no accident that many outdoor therapies originated in the field of experiential education. Clients in outdoor therapies may be engaged in structured adventure activities, extended expeditions in remote places, or in relationship with the land through cultural and historical practices. Regardless of the approach, active engagement in nature elicits responses from the body that play a meaningful role in the therapeutic process (Shanahan, Franco, Lin, Gaston, & Fuller, 2016).

The outdoors can be an ideal setting for one's learning of inner and outer landscapes. Client sensory awareness can be heightened (Harper, Rose, & Segal, 2019), and physiological and emotional regulation (see Chapter 11) can be practiced and improved (Kain & Terrell, 2018). Physical activities in the outdoors are a dynamic process: Eyes adjust to changes in available light, breathing changes relative to hiking uphill or over challenging terrain, and our sense of balance adapts as we float or submerge ourselves in the ocean.

We remind readers that we do not promote nature as a panacea. During inclement weather or in difficult terrain, attention can be drained, and fatigue and stress can be magnified. The therapeutic calculus of outdoor therapies depends on the relation between a client's resources, the level of challenge, and the meaning derived from the experience. While it may be assumed we would avoid adverse conditions, some outdoor therapy approaches intentionally engage with weather, terrain, intensity, and remoteness based on the therapeutic goals of the client or group (Harper et al., 2019).

Outdoor Therapies Recognize Nature-Human Kinship

There is a third common element of outdoor therapies: The human-nature relationship. The outdoor therapists in this volume agree, depending on their relative embrace of holism, that we are 'part' of nature or simply 'are' nature. To go outdoors moves us closer to ourselves. As forest biology professor Robbin Wall-Kimmerer (2013), of the Citizen Potawatomi Nation, reminds us, 'kinship' between all living things has "the enduring power that arises from mutualism, from the sharing of gifts carried by each species" (p. 275).

The human experience of nature is diverse: Environmental refugees forced into overland migration on foot, children growing up isolated from nature in urban living conditions with the inability to see stars at night, naturalists—Indigenous and modern—who develop wisdom for the nuance and interplay of humans and other species. We recognize that a spectrum of human-nature connection is present. Outdoor therapies can be especially therapeutic for those who have become functionally and conceptually disconnected from nature, due to technological changes, urbanization, colonization, environmental devastation, and other socio-political forces. Outdoor therapies aim to address the disconnect and return vitality to humans as a species dependent upon the health of the planet for their own well-being.

In short, we are all nature and benefit immensely from this recognition and our ability to hold ourselves accountable to it. This is in contrast to a common human-centric understanding, as in the Oxford Dictionary and Wikipedia, that defines *nature* as "other than human." This perpetuates a dichotomy between humans, the physical world of plants and animals, and features of the Earth such as beaches, mountains, and rivers. Our collective experience and belief is that the fulfillment of one's potential is realized through a deep meaningful relationship and *inter-being* with nature, a revitalizing and normalizing of kinship with all living things. To bring our therapeutic work into relationship with the environment which sustains us seems the reasonable thing to do.

Compatibility for Outdoor Therapies

Who is best suited to receive the benefits of outdoor therapies? This question is relevant for both clients and practitioners. We know from our own experiences that to effectively engage in outdoor therapies, the practitioner's relationship with nature must come first. This need for a self-assessment is no different from training in any new modality. In the case of outdoor therapies, practitioners must develop their own nature awareness and ecological identity (Harper et al., 2019). Further, from a practical and risk management standpoint, you can reflect on what knowledge or skills you need to meaningfully engage clients outside of the office or facility that you work in.

For clients: What outdoor activities are you drawn to, and how do they conform to your values and needs for restoration and growth? What level of challenge and intensity seems appropriate? What knowledge, skills, and tools do you require? These questions help reveal what type of outdoor therapy might be most helpful for you. We propose a precautionary and thoughtful approach to answering these questions. A considered, professional assessment of both therapist and client needs and preferences related to the type, location, and intensity of outdoor therapy is required (see Hooley, 2016).

An Invitation to Walk

One of the most readily available outdoor practices for an office-based counselor or psychotherapist is to simply step outside and walk with their client (McKinney, 2011; Revell & McLeod, 2016). The 'walk and talk' mode had existed since modern psychotherapy began, and in many ways can be considered a 'gateway' to more integrative outdoor thera-peutic practices (Doucette, 2004). We are excited to hear of therapists taking this first step; incorporating an active, outdoor, lived-body expe-rience with their clients (Schwenk, 2019). At the same time, we acknowl-edge that many therapists have been practicing outdoors for years. We make no assumptions about the training, knowledge, and skills of our readers. Despite growing awareness and recognition of outdoor ther-apies, a review of counseling psychology training programs' inclusion of ecopsychology across the United States found few available course materials (Hoover & Slagle, 2015). Considering the well-known health benefits and broadened clinical outcomes associated with taking therapy outdoors, we strongly encourage mental health professionals to learn about and engage in these practices.

References

Annerstedt, M., & Währborg, P. (2011). Nature-assisted therapy: Systematic re-view of controlled and observational studies. *Scandinavian Journal of Public Health*, 39(4), 371–388.

Barnes, M. R., Donahue, M. L., Keeler, B. L., Shorb, C. M., Mohtadi, T. Z., & Shelby, L. J. (2019). Characterizing nature and participant experience in stud-ies of nature exposure for positive mental health, an integrative review. *Fron-tiers in Psychology*, 9, 2617.

Bélanger, M., Gallant, F., Doré, I., O'Loughlin, J. L., Sylvestre, M. P., Nader, P. A., ... & Sabiston, C. (2019). Physical activity mediates the relationship between outdoor time and mental health. *Preventive Medicine Reports*. doi:10.1016/j.pmedr.2019.101006

Berman, M. G., Kross, E., Krpan, K. M., Askren, M. K., Burson, A., Deldin, P. J., ... & Jonides, J. (2012). Interacting with nature improves cognition and affect for individuals with depression. *Journal of Affective Disorders*, 140(3), 300–305.

Berman, M. G., Stier, A. J., & Akcelik, G. N. (2019). Environmental neurosci-ence. *American Psychologist*, 74, 1039–1052.

Burls, A. (2007). People and green spaces: Promoting public health and mental well-being through ecotherapy. *Journal of Public Mental Health*, 6(3), 24–39.

Chandler, M. J., & Lalonde, C. (1998). Cultural continuity as a hedge against suicide in Canada's First Nations. *Transcultural Psychiatry*, 35(2), 191–219.

Corazon, S. S., Schilhab, T. S., & Stigsdotter, U. K. (2011). Developing the therapeutic potential of embodied cognition and metaphors in nature-based therapy: Lessons from theory to practice. *Journal of Adventure Education & Outdoor Learning*, 11(2), 161–171.

Doherty, T. J. (2016). Theoretical and empirical foundations for ecotherapy. In M. Jordan & J. Hinds (Eds.), *Ecotherapy: Theory, research & practice*. London, England: Palgrave.

Doherty, T. J. & Chen, A. (2016). Improving human functioning: Ecotherapy and environmental health approaches. In R. Gifford (Ed.), *Research methods in envi-ronmental psychology*. (pp. 323–343), Hoboken, NJ: John Wiley & Sons.

Doherty, T. J., & Clayton, S. (2011). The psychological impacts of global climate change. *American Psychologist, 66*(4), 265–276.

Doucette, P. A. (2004). Walk and talk: An intervention for behaviorally challenged youths. *Adolescence, 39*(154), 373–388.

Duncan, M. J., Vandelanotte, C., Caperchione, C., Hanley, C., & Mummery, W. K. (2012). Temporal trends in and relationships between screen time, physical activity, overweight and obesity. *BMC Public Health, 12*(1), 1060.

Fernee, C. R., Gabrielsen, L. E., Andersen, A. J., & Mesel, T. (2017). Unpacking the black box of wilderness therapy: A realist synthesis. *Qualitative Health Research, 27*(1), 114–129.

Fritze, J. G., Blashki, G. A., Burke, S., & Wiseman, J. (2008). Hope, despair and transformation: Climate change and the promotion of mental health and wellbeing. *International Journal of Mental Health Systems, 2*(1), 13.

Gabrielsen, L. E., & Harper, N. J. (2018). The role of wilderness therapy for adolescents in the face of global trends of urbanization and technification. *International Journal of Adolescence and Youth, 23*(4), 409–421.

Garcia, J. A. & Weisz, J. R. (2002). When youth mental health care stops: Therapeutic relationship problems and other reasons for ending youth outpatient treatment. *Journal of Consulting & Clinical Psychology, 70*(2), 439–443.

Geronimus, A. T., Bound, J., Waidmann, T. A., Rodriguez, J. M., & Timpe, B. (2019). Weathering, drugs, and whack-a-mole: Fundamental and proximate causes of widening educational inequity in US life expectancy by sex and race, 1990–2015. *Journal of Health and Social Behavior, 60*(2), 222–239.

Harper, C., Harper, C. L., & Snowden, M. (2017). *Environment and society: Human perspectives on environmental issues.* New York, NY: Routledge.

Harper, N. J., Rose, K., & Segal, D. (2019). *Nature-based therapy: A practitioner's guide to working outdoors with children, youth, and families.* Gabriola Island, Canada: New Society Publishers.

Hooley, I. (2016). Ethical considerations for psychotherapy in natural settings. *Ecopsychology, 8*(4), 215–221.

Hoover, S. M., & Slagle, C. P. (2015). A preliminary assessment of ecopsychology education in counseling psychology doctoral training programs. *Ecopsychology, 7*(3), 160–165.

Jiang, B., Chang, C. Y., & Sullivan, W. C. (2014). A dose of nature: Tree cover, stress reduction, and gender differences. *Landscape and Urban Planning, 132*, 26–36.

Jordan, M., & Marshall, H. (2010). Taking counselling and psychotherapy outside: Destruction or enrichment of the therapeutic frame? *European Journal of Psychotherapy & Counselling, 12*, 345–359.

Kain, K. L., & Terrell, S. J. (2018). *Nurturing resilience.* Berkeley, CA: North Atlantic Books.

Kaplan, S., & Berman, M. G. (2010). Directed attention as a common resource for executive functioning and self-regulation. *Perspectives on Psychological Science, 5*(1), 43–57.

Kellert, S. R., & Wilson, E. O. (Eds.). (1995). *The biophilia hypothesis.* Washington, DC: Island Press.

Kimmerer, R. (2013). *Braiding sweetgrass: Indigenous wisdom, scientific knowledge and the teachings of plants.* Minneapolis, MN: Milkweed Editions.

Klepeis, N. E., Nelson, W. C., Ott, W. R., Robinson, J. P., Tsang, A. M., Switzer, P., ... & Engelmann, W. H. (2001). The National Human Activity Pattern Survey (NHAPS): A resource for assessing exposure to environmental pollutants. *Journal of Exposure Science and Environmental Epidemiology*, *11*(3), 231–252.

Kondo, M. C., South, E. C., & Branas, C. C. (2015). Nature-based strategies for improving urban health and safety. *Journal of Urban Health*, *92*(5), 800–814.

Kontis, V., Bennett, J. E., Mathers, C. D., Li, G., Foreman, K., & Ezzati, M. (2017). Future life expectancy in 35 industrialised countries: Projections with a Bayesian model ensemble. *The Lancet*, *389*(10076), 1323–1335.

Lavallee, L. F., & Poole, J. M. (2010). Beyond recovery: Colonization, health and healing for Indigenous people in Canada. *International Journal of Mental Health and Addiction*, *8*(2), 271–281.

Li, Q. (2010). Effect of forest bathing trips on human immune function. *Environmental Health and Preventive Medicine*, *15*(1), 9.

Maller, C., Townsend, M., Pryor, A., Brown, P., & St. Leger, L. (2005). Healthy nature healthy people: 'contact with nature' as an upstream health promotion intervention for populations. *Health Promotion International*, *21*(1), 45–54.

McKinney, B. L. (2011). Therapist's perceptions of walk and talk therapy: A grounded study. Unpublished Doctoral Dissertation. Lafayette: University of Louisiana.

Merikangas, K. R., He, J. P., Burstein, M., Swanson, S. A., Avenevoli, S., Cui, L., ... & Swendsen, J. (2010). Lifetime prevalence of mental disorders in US adolescents: Results from the National Comorbidity Survey Replication–Adolescent Supplement (NCS-A). *Journal of the American Academy of Child & Adolescent Psychiatry*, *49*(10), 980–989.

Moodley, R., & West, W. (Eds.). (2005). *Integrating traditional healing practices into counseling and psychotherapy* (Vol. 22). Thousand Oaks, CA: Sage.

Mygind, L., Kjeldsted, E., Dalgaard Hartmeyer, R., Mygind, E., Bølling, M., & Bentsen, P. (2019). Immersive nature-experiences as health promotion interventions for healthy, vulnerable, and sick populations? A systematic review and appraisal of controlled studies. *Frontiers in Psychology*, *10*, 943.

Neumann, A., Ojong, T. N., Yanes, P. K., Tumiel-Berhalter, L., Daigler, G. E., & Blondell, R. D. (2010). Differences between adolescents who complete and fail to complete residential substance abuse treatment. *Journal of Addictive Diseases*, *29*(4), 427–435.

Norwood, M. F., Lakhani, A., Fullagar, S., Maujean, A., Downes, M., Byrne, J., ... & Kendall, E. (2019). A narrative and systematic review of the behavioural, cognitive and emotional effects of passive nature exposure on young people: Evidence for prescribing change. *Landscape and Urban Planning*, *189*, 71–79.

Pasanen, T. P., Tyrväinen, L., & Korpela, K. M. (2014). The relationship between perceived health and physical activity indoors, outdoors in built environments, and outdoors in nature. *Applied Psychology: Health and Well-Being*, *6*(3), 324–346.

Poitras, V. J., Gray, C. E., Borghese, M. M., Carson, V., Chaput, J. P., Janssen, I., ... & Sampson, M. (2016). Systematic review of the relationships between objectively measured physical activity and health indicators in school-aged children and youth. *Applied Physiology, Nutrition, and Metabolism*, *41*(6), S197–S239.

Revell, S., & McLeod, J. (2016). Experiences of therapists who integrate walk and talk into their professional practice. *Counselling and Psychotherapy Research*, 16(1), 35–43.

Richards, K., Hardie, A., & Anderson, N. (2019). *Outdoor mental health interventions. Institute for Outdoor Learning statement of good practice.* Carlisle, England: Institute for Outdoor Learning.

Robbins, J. A., & Dewar, J. (2011). Traditional Indigenous approaches to healing and the modern welfare of traditional knowledge, spirituality and lands: A critical reflection on practices and policies taken from the Canadian Indigenous example. *The International Indigenous Policy Journal*, 2(4), 2.

Schwenk, H. (2019). Outdoor therapy: An interpretative phenomenological analysis examining the lived-experience, embodied, and therapeutic process through interpersonal process recall. *Sports*, 7(8), 182.

Shanahan, D. F., Astell–Burt, T., Barber, E. A., Brymer, E., Cox, D. T., Dean, J., ... & Jones, A. (2019). Nature-based interventions for improving health and wellbeing: The purpose, the people and the outcomes. *Sports*, 7(6), 141.

Shanahan, D. F., Franco, L., Lin, B. B., Gaston, K. J., & Fuller, R. A. (2016). The benefits of natural environments for physical activity. *Sports Medicine*, 46(7), 989–995.

Silove, D., Ventevogel, P., & Rees, S. (2017). The contemporary refugee crisis: An overview of mental health challenges. *World Psychiatry*, 16(2), 130–139.

Smith, L. T., Tuck, E., & Yang, K. W. (Eds.). (2019). *Indigenous and decolonizing studies in education.* New York, NY: Routledge.

Taylor, A. F., & Kuo, F. E. (2009). Children with attention deficits concentrate better after walk in the park. *Journal of Attention Disorders*, 12(5), 402.

Toffler, A. (1984). *Future shock* (Vol. 553). New York, NY: Bantam.

Twine, F. W., & Gardener, B. (Eds.). (2013). *Geographies of privilege.* New York, NY: Routledge.

United Nations. (2018). Revision of the world urbanization prospects. Department of Economic and Social Affairs. Retrieved December 3, 2019 from https://www.un.org/development/desa/publications/2018-revision-of-world-urbanization-prospects.html

White, L. (1967). The historical roots of our ecologic crisis. *Science*, 155, 1203–1207.

Wildcat, M., McDonald, M., Irlbacher-Fox, S., & Coulthard, G. (2014). Learning from the land: Indigenous land based pedagogy and decolonization. *Decolonization: Indigeneity, Education & Society*, 3(3), 1–15.

Wilmot, E. G., Edwardson, C. L., Achana, F. A., Davies, M. J., Gorely, T., Gray, L. J., ... & Biddle, S. J. H. (2012). Sedentary time in adults and the association with diabetes, cardiovascular disease and death: Systematic review and meta-analysis. *Diabetologia*, 55, 2895–2905.

Wilson, N., Ross, M., Lafferty, K., & Jones, R. (2009). A review of ecotherapy as an adjunct form of treatment for those who use mental health services. *Journal of Public Mental Health*, 7(3), 23–35.

Wolsko, C., & Lindberg., K. (2013). Experiencing connection with nature: The matrix of psychological well-being, mindfulness, and outdoor recreation. *Ecopsychology*, 5(2), 80–91.

Chapter 2

Experiential Facilitation in the Outdoors

Luk Peeters and Martin Ringer

Introduction and Background

This chapter addresses some of the history and cultural perspectives of the therapeutic facilitation of outdoor endeavors. We think that modern-day 'experiential therapies' are in part an attempt to recover cultural wisdom that has been lost from Western society and more recently also from Indigenous cultures. With the increasing reliance on theories, techniques, and methods, we risk forgetting that learning from one's own experience is a fundamental human capability, based on the three following competencies: (1) The ability to notice the consequences of one's actions and inactions in relation to the actual needs of one's environment; (2) the capacity to take in relevant information from one's own perception and experience, from other peoples' opinions and from the other-than-human surroundings that can be used to develop learning; and (3) the capacity to manage one's own feelings and thoughts well enough to integrate the learning that arises from the above—rather than avoiding acknowledging one's central role in one's own experience.

Nonetheless, traumatic events or episodes can endanger or disturb (temporarily) the capacity for self-healing, even if a specific person or a culture has access to a well-developed and attentive experiential noticing and processing system (Ginot, 2015). Even without the effect of trauma, one might block their own awareness and experiencing in a specific situation because of a need for emotional or psychological survival. It is in the circumstances where people have lost their innate capacity of learning from their own experience that facilitation from 'the other' might be necessary or needed, in order to restore the self-healing capacity.

The theoretical underpinning and practices of outdoor therapies are influenced by mainly two fields: Experiential and process-oriented therapies and outdoor education (Harper, Peeters, & Carpenter, 2015). Experiential therapies and process-oriented treatments, such as Gestalt (Perls, Hefferline, & Goodman, 1951), person-centered (Rogers, 1961), focusing (Gendlin, 1978), bioenergetic analysis (Lowen, 1958), and psychodrama (Moreno, 1946), can be observed in outdoor therapies. These approaches were influenced in their development by existential and phenomenological philosophies, the development of psychoanalytic schools of thought, and Eastern religions. The outdoor (experiential) educational movement had theoretical and philosophical roots in the work of people such as Dewey (1938) for experience and education, Kolb (1984) for experience and learning styles, Hahn (Schwarz, 1968) for outdoor adventure, Piaget (1972) for developmental theory and constructivist theory of knowing, Freire (1968) for emancipatory education, and from Illich's (1971) criticisms of formal education. However as outdoor therapies evolve, it seems that therapeutic approaches and belief-systems grow with increasing cross-fertilization between disciplines. In our view, this brief, and quite likely incomplete overview of contributors, illustrates the richness of theoretical influences which provide diverse potential and surprising innovation in our work.

Adventure therapy (see Chapter 7) has evolved from a model where it was thought that the activity could speak for itself (Bacon, 1987) through to a model influenced by other humanistic disciplines, and that reflection upon the activity is a necessary therapeutic element (Gass & Priest, 2005). In a further elaboration of theory, the deliberate use of metaphor and frontloading techniques was advocated, which drew attention to the presentation, or the briefing of the activity or encounter that was to follow (Bacon, 1983; Gass, Gillis, & Priest, 2000). More recently, we have arrived at models that transcend earlier linear simplifications of well-known and commonly used learning cycles (Hovelynck, 2000; Kolb, 1984). These ideas emphasize more of a reflection-in-action approach where the meaning-making process of the participants is the focus of our facilitation attention, during *every* element of the program. That is, it is important to not distinguish between the phases of presentation, briefing, action, reflection, and transfer. Rather, participant learning emerges from a holistic and integrated process of facilitation throughout the entire duration of participants engagements with the therapeutic program.

Concepts and Paradigms

We distinguish between experiential outdoor approaches and other outdoor processes that are not grounded in *experiencing*. These other approaches, such as narrative-based adventure therapy or cognitive behavioral-based adventure therapy, are an essential part of the whole ecology of outdoor-based learning and therapy (Gass, Gillis, & Russell, 2012). However, the facilitation of depth-based outdoor experiential learning focuses more on the experiencing as a whole, which is a complex interplay of emotion, different kinds of memory, cognition, bodily awareness, action, needs, and motivation (Greenberg, Watson, & Lietaer, 1998). It also calls on us to explore some of the undercurrents in individuals and groups that are often overlooked in other approaches (Ringer, 2002), which usually occur outside the direct awareness of both participants and facilitators (Peeters & Ringer, 2015).

For many years, practitioners, largely from outside the outdoor field, have been refining therapeutic systems that take into account unconscious processes, systems dynamics, and personal and group dynamics (Huckabay, 1992; Taylor, Segal, & Harper, 2010). We draw on these to help inform our practice as outdoor therapeutic practitioners and make some broad generalizations referring to the use of *self-as-instrument*, of which we will expand on later in this chapter.

Experiential therapeutic approaches view people as experiencing agents who, by symbolizing and reflecting on their experience, construct new meaning and choose courses of action (Greenberg et al., 1998). This belief holds the paradigm that the individual is the specialist of their own situation and that we potentially possess the best possible responses to deal with the questions and challenges that we have to face in our own personal lives. What we are aware of and what we feel, our thoughts and emotions, are herein the best guidelines we have at our disposal.

About Limits, Boundaries, and Blockages to Experiencing Change

A central concept in the change process is awareness. The paradoxical theory of change describes how we must get acquainted with our dysfunctional ways of being through fully engaging with all of our awareness (Beisser, 1970; Philippson, 2012). It is the process of a heightened awareness that will logically, but inevitably, lead to change. Having said that, being immersed in an activity does not necessarily mean that we will *experience* it. In that sense, we find it confusing and misleading that some literature (e.g., Gass et al., 2012) does not make any differentiation between a proposed activity or program component, and the idiosyncratic experiences that these might evoke in different participants. To us, this is not a mere question of semantics. There is a huge difference between what is offered or what we engage people in (action or activity) and how this is perceived. Participant's unique and personal experience varies greatly, depending on what sensations, images, metaphors, feelings, and thoughts are provoked and evoked. We want to strongly affirm that in our view we cannot provide experiences. We can only provide occasions, or an environment, or encounters that may generate experiences that can be worked with by engaging with each participant's experience.

The core of the difficulty is that we often act out of habit, unconscious beliefs, or outdated emotional schema's (Peeters, 2003). These are developed earlier in life in response to perceived threat or danger in the environment at the time, but repeated later in life, even when they are no longer an appropriate response to the current environment (Greenberg, Rice, & Elliot, 1993). For example, repeated experiences with punitive teachers might have influenced a reaction to back off and shy away in situations where we encounter authority figures, even if, for example, our new boss is positive minded and open to disagreement.

People develop strategies which can block their own awareness, especially in novel or potentially emotional overwhelming situations or when focused on a goal or task completion. For example, if we want to finish a hike it is better not to feel a developing blister. To be able to get up onto the horse's back, it is not helpful to be aware of the growing fear inside of you. Perhaps too, if there is a social or cultural norm that forbids being emotional, it is better not to feel the upcoming sadness.

Thanks to developments in the fields of neuroscience, neuropsychology, and social neuroscience, we now understand that the brain, mind, and body are an interrelated system and that our sense of 'self' as being separate from 'other' is largely an illusion (Biran, 2015; Ginot, 2015). This discussion is expanded on in Chapter 11 about sensory integrated occupational therapy in the outdoors. There is also considerable evidence that the majority of our significant emotional and psychological events, and learning, occur outside our conscious awareness (Ginot, 2015; Wilson, 2004). This leads to the notion that it is no longer possible for facilitators to see ourselves as separate from the group we facilitate. We are immersed in a complex manifestation of conscious and unconscious processes that involves our own emotional and psychological worlds at least as much as it does those of our participants.

Experiential Facilitation Outdoors

The Latin origins of the word facilitate is facilis; to make easier. The central task of the facilitation process is to 'ease' the self-development and healing process of the client. We cannot provide learning or healing ourselves. We need to nurture its presence in the client. Perhaps a suitable metaphor for the role of the facilitator is that of a blind guide who is going to lead someone (the client) through a territory that is unknown to both. The guide has to rely on the sight of the client to identify a safe route that enables safe travel through the area. By asking questions and assisting the client to look differently or at particular features of the landscape, they succeed together in passing many obstacles and finding a route that leads them through. The guide assists with the traveler (client) experience in route-finding and by their ability to read the landscape. The guide also discusses with the traveler the significance of the different features in this particular environment.

As argued before, it is the client or participant that is the expert on their own life; making sense of purpose and direction themselves. Facilitating will thus start from this frame of reference and from the experienced world of the client. This means that facilitation of outdoor therapies is an emergent process rather than one that can follow procedures, routines, and methods. There are no *how-to's* applicable to all situations. Fortunately, we are not entirely lost in the unknowable. We can identify some skills and capacities that are likely to be helpful to facilitators in many situations, and these are outlined in the following sections.

Focus on purpose is a key element: The ever-present reflective question is: "Are there any signs that the individuals or the group are experiencing something useful at that very moment?" Furthermore, "What might that be?" These are very different from the more common questions facilitators ask themselves, such as "Is the activity going to plan?"

A second key attitude is to consider yourself as a sensory 'emotional radar' for what is going on in the group. For example, it may seem that things are going well in a particular moment but the practitioner becomes aware of strong tinges of sadness. If there is nothing in his/her awareness that would normally make one sad, it is well worth asking oneself if they are picking up this sadness from individuals or the group. This self-as-instrument attitude helps practitioners to be comfortable with the idea that facilitation is a constant negotiation between group, individuals, the environment, and the facilitator. Everything can change in a moment.

The Therapeutic Relationship

The therapeutic relationship between therapist/facilitator and client/participant is key in facilitating exploration, risk-taking, experimentation, insight, and change (Greenberg et al., 1998; O'Brien, 1990). The genuine and authentic relationship is mainly established, maintained, and sometimes even restored by a participant's experience of a practitioner's empathy, acceptance, and congruence (Elliot, Watson, Goldman, & Greenberg, 2003). The very presence of a therapist who can stay present with, in contact with, and attuned to participants is a strong positive therapeutic element. For this to happen, therapists need to stay connected with themselves and with their participants even when there are strong currents of difficult emotion involved (Ringer, 2017).

Heightening the Awareness and the Process Capacity of Participants

As stated earlier, the process of heightening awareness is considered to be one of the keys to change. Already, the novel environment of outdoor therapy might in itself heighten the *here-and-now* awareness of the participant (Peeters, 2015). Participants perhaps experience themselves being more fully present and alive, feeling outside sensations such as the wind, the smells, or the temperature, whilst at the same time noticing their own heart-rate, heavy breathing, shivering or blushing. The practical demands of the unfamiliar setting might also contrast very much with our habitual but-not-so-functional patterns and might make them suddenly visible. A participant describes how his delaying and hesitating coping-style became very obvious and hindering when he had to choose between three passages in a caving situation. He became cold and wet, suffering his inability to make a choice. Facilitators can assist participants adding to this heightening of awareness process.

Taking a Process-Oriented Stance

As mentioned before, a focus on the completion of a 'task' or an assignment might block, numb, or hinder the process of being fully in the here-and-now. The local expression "with your eyes on infinity and your brain on zero you can overcome any challenge" describes this well.

Instead of presenting the objective of the activity in terms of tasks-results, such as to stand on top of the pole, to get on the back of the horse, or to find the second exit of the cave, we advocate for a shift toward a process-oriented framework. Perhaps with wording like "try to notice what happens to you as you move up toward and perhaps on to that pole." This moves the stated goal from task success to make room for the personal objectives of participants to be realized (Hovelynck, 1999).

It could be a much bigger success for a participant in the framework of personal growth and healing to deliberately not participate in a group activity instead of the well-known coping style of doing what the rest of the group members do, whatever negative consequences that might bring to the individual participant. For example, in reflecting over a caving activity, a participant of a psychotherapy training group shares that she is very proud that she actually did not enter the cave and decided at the entrance to walk back on her own to the center where they were staying.

> I know myself as someone very competitive, never yielding in the presence of others. Often realizing that I do not find any joy in doing those things, only wanting to show that I too am capable of it. So, I feel proud now, I chose for myself, for my own comfort and benefit and I can even listen to your wonderful cave stories without any frustration or sadness or putting myself down. This is a big realization for me.

Establishing and Maintaining a Reflective Space

Peeters (2003) and Ringer (2002) stressed the importance of creating a psychologically supportive atmosphere and environment that facilitates awareness, curiosity, and eagerness in exploring and sharing one's own internal processes. Not only does this provide, in a passive way, the necessary safety, it also actively engages everyone to share a fascinating journey of discovery. This reflective space is built through the role-modeling of the facilitator and the collaborative establishing of norms that support the above, for example, being comfortable with long silences, and disclosing personal feelings if they seem related to the life of the group at the moment.

Naming of Activities or Tasks

The name we give an activity and how it is described to participants might narrow or block potential awareness during the subsequent activity. For example, calling an activity a 'trust fall,' 'pamper-pole,' or a 'death-ride' strongly suggests where the facilitators expect your awareness to go. So, we prefer names that are more descriptive in nature like 'backward fall,' 'high pole,' or 'the pulley descent.'

Even so, we should ensure that the focus is not drawn toward completion of what might be suggested in the name, but rather on getting involved in a relationship with self-in-process. A facilitator might describe an activity as follows:

> This high pole might be explored in different ways. Some people climb it and try to notice what it does to them or how they relate with the people holding their safety line, for instance. Other people try to climb up, to stand on it, and jump off. Others may see it as an occasion to go against the flow, or sensing the performance-pressure they notice from themselves or the group, choose not to climb. Or perhaps you can think of another approach that might suit your needs even better.

Tailor-Make Your 'Encounters' and Grade Them Accordingly

In the same way, we suggest creating activities that are related as much as possible to the idiosyncratic needs of every participant. Such activities can be tailor-made in terms of intensity so as to meet the participants 'level of readiness' to engage (Peeters, 2015; Zinker, 1977). This helps the client to execute an experiment at the level which they are ready to do so in a given context. Note that the use of 'experiment' in our context does not have the same meaning as in the classic scientific setting. Within this context, it is the acceptance of a challenge, the willingness to try something new, and being curious about the outcome. Adjustment of the level of intensity for an activity should be done, not only to meet the level of readiness of the participant, but also to take into account surrounding circumstances, such as the length of the program and group dynamic mechanisms.

Standard adventure activities can be engaged in at a personalized level for each participant (Peeters, 2003). Moreover, even the refusal of getting involved in what is presented can be regarded as a success if that coping style can be processed and explored. Hence, 'success' in an activity for a participant is not completion of the task, but rather engaging emotionally with the task, and being able to reflect on and learn from their actions or inactions. For example, a group is invited to take 12 hours of solo time, each at a separate spot during a mountain journey. On hearing the proposal, one participant immediately tells the therapist and the group that he will not go. He talks in a very emotional and engaged way, sharing that he has had a very painful history of solitude and being on his own, feeling very clumsy in social contacts and having developed a distrust in others. During the program, he developed some trust and gained confidence in relating to others. He is afraid that for him this invitation comes too prematurely and that even imagining to be separated from the people he just started to like and trust would feel terrifying. Then he sighs saying, "What a relief to be able to share this with all of you. It seems that I already gained a lot from my solo time!"

Intervene Actively

We should actively engage ourselves as facilitators in every phase of the program to process-direct the exploration of a potential growing awareness. In experiential facilitation, we are not non-directive, nor are we product-directive. We do no direct participants toward certain outcomes, but rather direct them where and how to place their attention. We avoid telling them what to see, we tell them where to look, and then we ask them what they see.

During the activities, we can assist in a growing awareness by restricting sensory input. For example, we can suggest a client to continue the rock-climbing with her eyes closed and explore for herself the similarities and differences she is aware of. We can ask for silence and use a soft tone ourselves to limit possible distracting sensations. We can ask a participant to stop the action, pause, and turn the attention inside toward bodily sensations, feelings, and recurring thoughts. We can also invite someone to repeat a specific action and even ask them to exaggerate it.

We can openly share our observations. For example, we might say to a participant: "You say you do not want to approach the horse and at the same time I see your feet moving in that direction." We can even imitate certain features (body movements, sighs, groans, etc.) to facilitate awareness and further meaning-making. This can reflect unconscious material that escapes the awareness of the participant and enables the participant to engage more fully with their experience in the moment. An example is of a facilitator that imitates the participant saying "I know," whilst sighing loudly and looking down. The participant reacts saying, "Oh I see, so that is what I do when I say I know. Yes, I sometimes feel hopeless wondering if I will ever be capable of changing, yet I want so dearly to be different."

Those interventions do not have to be limited to the physical action-phase of the program. During the introduction of a caving activity, the facilitator suddenly notices, "Hey Linda, what is happening? I notice that you slowly started shaking your head." Linda then replies "Yes, it is that ugly competitive inner coach again who starts pushing me not to withdraw and not to show any weakness. Perhaps I am getting ready for an alternative approach." In the same sense, episodes that focus more on reflection are experiences as well and are not limited to 'data-processing' parts of an 'experiential learning' cycle.

The Strength of Embodied Metaphors

There is a long tradition in utilizing the strength of metaphor in psychotherapy, in general, and in outdoor therapies in particular (Bacon, 1983; Hartford, 2011; Hovelynck, 1999). Out of our general thinking about ownership and expertise, we try to avoid using pre-constructed metaphors. Rather than facilitator derived, we make space for and enhance metaphors that emerge from participant experiences. We are present and attentive to the way participants themselves make reference to images or figures, and we then build on these to enhance therapeutic outcomes. Participant words during activity, such as feeling supported or losing track, are often rooted in concrete behavior, and metaphors easily emerge and can be fully lived without having to be symbolically transformed.

Attention toward 'Wondering' or 'Immersion' in Contrast to 'Challenging'

Within this chapter, we also want to draw attention toward an aspect of being therapeutically present in an outdoor environment. This aspect of our work has received little attention in the literature of outdoor therapies; especially so in the more physically active outdoor therapies, such as wilderness therapy and adventure therapy. Being present is somewhat opposite to the aims of 'challenge,' 'endure,' 'strive,' 'risk-taking,' and 'conquering' found as elements of some outdoor therapies (Bacon, 1983). Being present is about immersing oneself in the beauty of the landscape or the environment, such as being overwhelmed by the silence, or the smells, or the colors, or the slowness and the graceful curves of the river.

Gently moving through the forest can be an act of meditative quality and can be facilitated to bring our participants truly into the here-and-now. Combined with a growing or renewed interest in stillness, seen in mindfulness and meditation offerings for mental health, in our thinking, is a major pathway to healing and toward more spiritual elements of the outdoor therapies as well as an area deserving far more attention than it has yet received (see Kirwin, Harper, Young, & Itzvan, 2019).

A group of participants who had been referred to an adventure therapy program because of repeated gang-related crime were sitting on the sand hills in the early evening after a long day of walking. As the sun started to dip below the horizon of the sea, there was an unusual silence in the group. The sun disappeared and a glorious show of color appeared in the clouds. Breaking the silence, a particularly staunch participant spoke with strong emotion "Wow man, that's Fuckin' choice!"

Working Alongside with 'Co-facilitators' and Utilizing Their Full Potential

What distinguishes outdoor therapies from more classical forms of therapy is the utilization of a special environment or activity. That environment may, as in the case of equine or animal-assisted therapy, include other living beings. Since a number of programs take place in a group context, the group itself is also considered to have therapeutic potential (Ringer, 2002). The task of the therapist is then to facilitate, to make it more easy, for those therapeutic elements to be utilized in their full potential.

For instance, a potential brilliant facilitator intervention might be less effective in the long term than a not-so-sophisticated well-meant comment from one participant to another, or a group-level invitation toward an individual. We strongly believe in the adage that if we take care of the group, the group will take care of its members (Foulkes & Anthony, 1957).

Nature as well needs the 'time' and 'space' to play its role. During one of the many uphill climbs on a multiday hiking program, a participant who survived cancer and had to deal with the passing-away of her husband in that same period yelled at the therapist that she was fed-up with the endless uphill walking. The last ten years had been a physical and emotional climb and she wanted some easy downhill walking now. "If I cannot come up with a mental reframing to deal with this I will not be able to continue this hike," she desperately shouted out. "I am here, close to you, and I will follow your pace" was the only thing the therapist answered. An hour later, on the top of the hill and enjoying the beautiful landscape below she turned again to the therapist, tired but with a smile. "I would never have been able to admire all of this without suffering the climb!" and then after a brief silence, "and I also realize that climbing up is the only way to get out of a deep, dark, and cold valley."

Tapping into the Not-Yet-Aware and the Unconscious: The Use of Self-as-Instrument

The structure of the brain means that some forms of learning and change occur directly through experience and are not accessible for verbal processing (Jansen & Pawson, 2015; Rae & Nichols, 2012). Neither participants nor facilitators have conscious awareness of all the learning that may be occurring. Nor do they have conscious access to some of the complex emotional undercurrents that occur in individuals or that circulate in groups. However, some of the complex emotional and psychological dynamics are made available as flashes of intuition or pervasive feelings. As a result, much of what we feel and experience emotionally as facilitators is a direct result of what is being felt and experienced by participants: We act as 'lightning rods' for participant's feelings, which often occurs outside our direct awareness, which some refer to as self-as-instrument (Hinshelwood, 2016). This leaves the uncomfortable question for facilitators, "But how do I know if what I am feeling is 'me' or coming from the group?" We can never be sure. If our feelings seem not to fit our expectations or seem unusual given the context, it is well worth considering that you are picking up feelings from group members.

The more we know about our habitual emotional responses, the greater the chance we will notice unusual feeling states. Hence, the more self-awareness facilitators have, the more likely they will be able to detect material useful to the participants (Foulkes & Anthony, 1957). Another element of using oneself as a therapeutic and facilitative instrument is our capacity to manage our own psychological and emotional equilibrium. When our "buttons are pushed," we need to be able to stay connected with ourselves and with our participants. This capacity can be developed with consistent personal work on the part of the facilitator and is a vital part of the therapeutic effectiveness of facilitators.

Conclusion

We hope we have provided the readers with some enthusiasm to consider the role of experiential facilitation in outdoor therapies as a collaborative effort and co-creation amongst all participants and elements involved in any program or intervention. The facilitator or therapist, the participant or client, the other group members and the group-as-a-whole if this applies, and the environment- or methodology-specific co-therapist (the rock-face, the landscape, the horse, the pebbles, etc.) all play potentially vital roles in the therapeutic process. With this reality, it is then incumbent upon the facilitator to remain present to, and engage with, all dynamics and possibilities in the experiential process.

References

Bacon, S. (1983). *The conscious use of metaphor in Outward Bound*. Denver, CO: Colorado Outward Bound School.

Bacon, S. (1987). *The evolution of the Outward Bound process*. Greenwich, England: Outward Bound USA.

Beisser, A. (1970). The paradoxical theory of change. In J. Fagan & I. L. Sheperd (Eds.), *Gestalt therapy now: Theory, techniques, applications* (pp. 77–80). Palo Alto, CA: Science and Behavior Books.

Biran, H. (2015). *The courage of simplicity: Essential ideas in the work of W. R. Bion*. London, England: Karnac.

Dewey, J. (1938). *Experience and education*. New York, NY: Kappa Delta Pi.

Elliot, R., Watson, J., Goldman, R., & Greenberg, L. (2003). *Learning emotion-focused therapy. The process-experiential approach to change*. Washington, DC: American Psychological Association.

Foulkes, S. H., & Anthony, E. J. (1957). *Group psychotherapy*. Baltimore, MD: Penguin books.

Freire, P. (1968). *Pedagogy of the oppressed*. London, England: The Continuum International Publishing Group.

Gass, M., Gillis, L., & Priest, S. (2000). *The essential elements of facilitation*, Tulsa, OK: Learning Unlimited.

Gass, M., Gillis, L., & Russell, K. (2012). *Adventure therapy. Theory, research and practice*. New York, NY: Routledge.

Gass, M. A., & Priest, S. (2005). *Effective leadership in adventure programming* (2nd ed.), Champaign, IL: Human Kinetics.

Gendlin, E. (1978). *Focusing*. New York, NY: Everest House.

Ginot, E. (2015). *The neuropsychology of the unconscious: Integrating brain and mind in psychotherapy*. New York, NY: W. W. Norton & Company.

Greenberg, L., Rice L., & Elliot, R. (1993). *Facilitating emotional change. The moment-by-moment process*. New York, NY: The Guilford Press.

Greenberg, L., Watson, J., & Lietaer, G. (1998). *Handbook of experiential psychotherapy*. New York, NY: The Guilford Press.

Harper, N. J., Peeters, L., & Carpenter, C. (2015). Adventure therapy. In R. Black & K. S. Bricker (Eds.), *Adventure programming and travel in the 21st century* (pp. 221–236). State College, PA: Venture Publishing.

Hartford, G. (2011). Practical implications for the development of applied metaphor in adventure therapy. *Journal of Adventure Education & Outdoor Learning, 11*(2), 145–160. doi:10.1080/14729679.2011.633383

Hinshelwood, R. D. (2016). *Countertransference and Alive Moments: Help or Hindrance*. London, England: Process Press Limited.

Hovelynck, J. (1999). Facilitating the development of generative metaphors: Re-emphasizing participants' guiding images. *Australian Journal of Outdoor Education, 4*(1), 12–24. doi:10.1007/BF03400705

Hovelynck, J. (2000). Recognising and exploring action-theories: A reflection-in-action approach to facilitating experiential learning. *Journal of Adventure Education and Outdoor Learning, 1*(1), 7–20. doi:10.1080/14729670085200031

Huckabay, M. A. (1992). An overview of the theory and practice of Gestalt group process. *Gestalt Therapy: Perspectives and Applications*, 303–330.

Illich, I. (1971). *Deschooling society*. London, England: Marion Boyons Publishers.

Jansen, C., & Pawson, P. (2015). Developing 'challenging' young people: Honouring their authentic story. In A. Pryor, C. Carpenter, C. Norton, & J. Kirchner (Eds.), *Emerging insights: Proceedings of the fifth international adventure therapy conference 2009* (pp. 121–132). Prague, Czechia: European Sciences & Arts Publishing.

Kirwin, M., Harper, N. J., Young, T., & Itzvan, I. (2019). Mindful adventures: A pilot study of the outward bound mindfulness program. *Journal of Outdoor and Environmental Education*, 22(1), 75–90. doi:10.1007/s42322-019-00031-9

Kolb, D. (1984). *Experiential learning*. Englewood Cliffs, NJ: Prentice Hall.

Lowen, A. (1958). *Language of the body. Physical dynamics of character structure*. Burlington, VT: Alexander Lowen Foundation.

Moreno, J. L. (1946). *Psychodrama*. New York, NY: Beacon House.

O'Brien, M. (1990). Northland wilderness experience: An experiential program for the youth of Taitokerau. Psychology Department, The University of Auckland, Auckland. ERIC Document Reproduction Service ED 372886.

Peeters, L. (2003). From adventure to therapy: Some necessary conditions to enhance the therapeutic outcomes of adventure programming. In K. Richards & B. Smith (Eds.), *Therapy within adventure* (pp. 127–138). Augsburg, Germany: ZIEL.

Peeters, L. (2015). Taking therapy into the outdoors: Why and when and how to do so. In C. Norton, C. Carpenter, & A. Pryor (Eds.), *Adventure therapy around the globe: International perspectives and diverse approaches*. Chicago, IL: Common Ground Publishing.

Peeters, L., & Ringer, M. (2015). The hidden adventure. Group projective identification in the practice of adventure therapy. In C. Norton, C. Carpenter, & A. Pryor (Eds.), *Adventure therapy around the globe. International perspectives and diverse Approaches* (pp. 595–607). Chicago, IL: Common Ground Publishing.

Perls, F., Hefferline, R., & Goodman, P. (1951). *Gestalt therapy. Excitement and growth in the human personality*. New York, NY: Dell Publishing.

Philippson, P. (2012). *Gestalt therapy: Roots and branches-collected papers*. New York, NY: Routledge.

Piaget, J. (1972). *Psychology and epistemology: Towards a theory of knowledge*. Urbana, IL: Viking Press.

Rae, P., & Nichols, A. V. (2012). The aboriginal outdoor recreation program: Connection with country, culture, family and community. In A. Pryor, C. Carpenter, C. Norton, & J. Kirchner (Eds.), *Emerging insights: Proceedings of the fifth international adventure conference 2009* (pp. 139–143). Prague, Czechia: European Sciences & Arts Publishing.

Ringer, M. (2002). *Group Action: The dynamics of groups in therapeutic, educational and corporate settings*. London, England: Jessica Kingsley Publishers.

Ringer, T. M. (2017). The therapy in human connections. Australian Association for Bush Adventure Therapy Forum. Candlebark School, Victoria.

Rogers, C. (1961). *On becoming a person*. London, England: Constable and Company.

Schwarz, K. (1968). *Die Kurzschulen Kurt Hahns*. Düsseldorf, Germany: A. Henn Verlag.

Taylor, D., Segal, D., & Harper, N. (2010). The ecology of adventure therapy: An integral systems approach to therapeutic change. *Ecopsychology, 2*(2), 77–83. doi:10.1089/eco.2010.0002

Wilson, T. (2004). *Strangers to ourselves: Discovering the adaptive unconscious*. Boston, MA: Harvard University Press.

Zinker, J. (1977). *Creative process in Gestalt therapy*. New York, NY: Vintage Books.

Chapter 3

Ecopsychological Approaches to Therapy

Megan E. Delaney

Introduction

Ecopsychology is the marriage of ecology and psychology forming a union that provides a framework for understanding the deep connection the human psyche has with the earth (Roszak, Gomes, & Kanner, 1995). This chapter outlines the historical development, theory, and efficacy of ecopsychology including key theorists and scholars of the movement and others who have added layers to its foundation. Also included in the chapter is an overview of ecotherapy, the clinical practice of ecopsychology, and the way in which mental health practitioners can incorporate the natural world into a model of human wellness. The case of Jenna, a client struggling with making sense of her anxiety and her connection to the natural world, is offered to illustrate the practice of ecotherapy and the healing potential of a reciprocal relationship with the natural world.

Theory, Research, and Efficacy

The human-and-nature connection has long been explored in religious, philosophical, and academic disciplines (Jordan & Hinds, 2016). German-born psychologist Erich Fromm (1973) fled Nazi Germany to come to America, first used the term *biophilia* to describe one's love of life and living systems. The *biophilia hypothesis* was introduced by Harvard biologist Edward O. Wilson (1984), suggesting that humans affiliate with other living things and the natural world for survival and mental and physical stability. Wilson described human dependence on the earth to provide food and water, the emotional bond and positive effect of nature, and the connections that people have to specific animals and places. Wilson and others have explored the coevolution and interconnectedness humans have with other living systems contributed to the growing environmental movement of the time (Krčmářová, 2009) and advanced the philosophical basis and principles of ecopsychology (Doherty & Clayton, 2011; Kahn & Hasbach, 2012).

Theodore Roszak (1992), a historian by training, began thinking beyond the scientific aspects of the environmental movement to conceptualize how the industrial revolution cut off human conscious from the natural world. Roszak believed that humans possessed what he called an *ecological unconscious,* or the core of the mind; an ecological ego, an ethical position primarily viewing the self and the planet as one; the understanding of a primal need for a reciprocal relationship with the natural world. As Theodore Roszak (1992) stated, "the needs of the planet are the needs of the person, the rights of the person are the rights of the planet" (p. 321). Roszak has been credited with coining the term *ecopsychology* and stated that its goal "is to bridge human culture's long-standing, historical gulf between the psychological and the ecological, to see the needs of the plant and the person as a continuum" (p. 14). Roszak, Gomes, and Kanner (1995) produced an anthology on ecopsychology, gathering scholars from multiple disciplines to explore and expound upon the connection of humans and nature. The authors in this anthology looked beyond just the human experience and explored the connection of the natural world to human development and psychological wellness, although they offered little which spoke to diversity or cross-cultural perspectives.

Roszak (1992) conceptualized ecopsychology as the intersectionality of the movement of environmentalism and the discipline of psychology. Environmentalism, as we know, is the movement addressing the scientific, political, and societal influences for the protection and conservation of the planet. Psychology is the study of mental and emotional processes of an individual, and psychotherapy, in the traditional sense, is the process where a therapist and client explore emotional difficulties and mental illnesses in order to achieve a greater sense of emotional well-being. Roszak et al. (1995) sought to redefine emotional well-being on a "personal and planetary" (p. 1) level and framed ecopsychology with the following eight guiding principles:

- The ecological unconscious is the core of all human minds, and repression of this unconscious causes mental health distress in an industrialized society.
- The ecological unconscious represents, in essence, a record of the living history of the universe.
- The goal of ecopsychology is to address the ecological unconscious mind and bring it into consciousness with the goal of healing the relationship of humans and the natural world.
- As with other therapies, ecopsychology holds the developmental period of childhood as critical space to experience the harmonious relationship of nature within their emerging sense of self.

- The ecological ego develops toward an ethical responsibility to the earth as critical as our responsibilities to one another.
- Ecopsychology rejects the attempt to dominate and yield power over the natural world, traits that drive humans to find ways to control nature. As such, ecopsychology aligns with ecofeminism, a movement that draws parallels with the oppression and exploitation of women with the attempt to subjugate the natural world.
- While ecopsychology is deeply rooted in rejection of over-industrialization at the peril of nature, it is not a movement of anti-progress and respects the technological progress of our species.
- Ecopsychology is, at its core, a *synergy* of the emotional well-being of the person and the health of the earth as such, the needs of the planet are the needs of the person, the rights of the person are the rights of the planet.

These critical tenets of ecopsychology provide the foundation for which scholars, researchers, clinicians, and others support and expand the movement for human connection/reconnection with nature.

Eco-Grief

A critical element of ecopsychology is the belief that humans experience psychological distress from the suffering of the earth. Conn (1995) wrote, "When the earth hurts, who responds?" (p. 156), contending that we are impacted both physically and emotionally by the health (or illness) of the planet. Around us and all over the world, forests are dying, storms and fires are raging, oceans rising, ice caps melting, and species are becoming extinct. Food insecurity and hunger are causing animals and people to become ill, and much of earth's fresh water is polluted. There are still groups of people, political movements, and powerful individuals, however, denying the impact of the climate crisis and that it is largely human caused (Jylhä & Akrami, 2015). Ecopsychologists contend that the ailing planet sits heavy on human minds, whether conscious or unconscious, and that the fragility and vulnerability of the planet creates a deep-rooted anxiety in people (Ojala, 2018). This eco-anxiety is a feeling bred from not knowing if the planet, which houses and sustains all living things, is able to support the growing demands and the continued exploitation of resources (Conn, 1995; Jordan & Hinds, 2016).

Biophobia

The growing separation of humans in the modern western lifestyle from meaningful connections to the earth has, for some, morphed further to fear, a term known as biophobia (White & Heerwagen, 1998). Biophobia has a long evolutionary history for humans and, like any form of anxiety, is the body's way of assessing the safety of a situation (Cozolino, 2014). Fear of predatory animals, spiders, and snakes, for example, was necessary in order to survive. Humans also needed to understand the severity of weather patterns, such as approaching storms, or seasons that brought flooding or drought, in order to take the necessary survival steps. Today, most people do not need to worry about death from a spider bite, yet some of these fears are hardwired for justifiable reasons. Severe weather can result in profound devastation. Wild animals suffering from dwindling habitats or fire, searching for food and shelter, are forced to come into contact with humans and domesticated pets. The combination of the grief of the dying earth and fear of its potential to cause harm has shifted many human's relationship with the natural world, albeit often subconsciously, with many retreating to the safety of controlled environments (White & Heerwagen, 1998).

Many of us have retreated inside, spending more time indoors than ever. Increasingly sedentary and indoor lifestyles have resulted in the average adult spending only 7% of their day outdoors, a significant decrease in the last few decades (Diffey, 2011). Aggregating these statistics, this means the majority of humans living in industrialized countries spend almost 339 days a year indoors. Researchers have found this growing disconnection between humans and the outdoors correlate with the increasing ailments, such as anxiety, attention deficit disorder, diabetes, and obesity (Torio, Encinosa, Berdahl, McCormick, & Simpson, 2015). Yet, evidence suggests that spending time in nature can have scientifically beneficial outcomes for human health and well-being (Bratman, Hamilton, Hahn, Daily, & Gross, 2015; Thorp, Owen, Neuhaus, & Dunstan, 2011). In particular, research supports a strong connection between spending time in nature and mental well-being (Bratman et al., 2015; Waller, 2009), increased concentration (Faber Taylor & Kuo, 2011), reduction of symptoms related to depression (Morrison & Gore, 2010), and rejuvenation from mental fatigue (Brymer, Cuddihy, & Sharma-Brymer, 2010). Maller, Henderson-Wilson, and Townsend (2009) found that being connected to nature can help people feel centered and calm, while experiencing less anxiety and depression.

It is important to note that nature, while glorious and potentially healing, is still wild. As with wild animals, that natural world must be respected and treated with deference. Humans can get lost, develop hyperthermia or hypothermia, become affected by rapid changes in weather, struck by lightning, drown in a flood or even a calm body of water, get bit, stung, or attacked by an animal, ingest a poisonous plant, or get infected by a tick-borne illness, to name a few. As with all relationships, one must know their own strengths and limitations and be as prepared as possible for the unknown. Of course, exploring one's relationship with the natural world is one way that humans can be in touch with their surroundings and, as much as possible, be prepared for any potential risks.

International, national, and grassroots efforts are underway to reconnect humans with their surroundings, tapping into the healing and restorative power of nature. Young environmental activists like Greta Thunberg, Autumn Peltier, and Bruno Rodriguez are championing the global movement for radical and immediate action to address the climate crisis. Local organizations, parks, and nature centers offer programming, lectures, guided hikes, and places for exploring the natural world. Physicians and pediatricians can now write prescriptions for spending time outdoors, intended to help patients and their families get outside (Carrell, 2018). Still widely unexplored, but gaining traction in different arenas, is the impact counselors, therapists, and psychologists can make to connect their clients with the healing power of nature by infusing it in the therapeutic process. The therapeutic work that encompasses the natural world is known as ecotherapy.

Discussion of Practice

At the same time that Roszak et al. (1995) were publishing their anthology on the topic of ecopsychology, Clinebell (1996) coined the term ecotherapy and conceptualized the work as a form of *ecological spirituality,* or a deeper connection to nature. In agreement with Roszak (1992), Clinebell felt that humans' relationship with the natural world must be mutually beneficial in that as nature has the capacity to heal people, people must also heal nature. Clinebell explained this reciprocity through his conceptualizing of the following three dimensions: *inreach, upreach,* and *outreach. Inreach* is the ability of humans to be nurtured by nature, intentionally permitting humans the capacity to experience and appreciate what the natural world offers us. *Upreach* expands upon that relationship with nature and allows humans to develop a more spiritual awareness, which in turn allows us to participate in *outreach,* or engagement in causes and actions that support and sustain the health and healing of the planet.

Building upon these concepts, scholars and ecotherapists have contributed additional nuances to the ideas of ecopsychology and ecotherapy. Buzzell and Chalquist (2009) offered *green psychology* in the form of questions, techniques, and curiosities. The authors presented ways in which therapists can start incorporating ecotherapy within different conventional modalities. For example, consider the clinicians' awakening of their own human-nature connection, and how this emerging understanding can begin to influence their work as therapists. The authors shared the inclusion of ecotherapy principles across differing populations, places, and issues.

Ecotherapy is often referred to as applied ecopsychology, and eco-therapists utilize various techniques and interventions to emphasize the reciprocal relationship of humans and nature (Jordan & Hinds, 2016). Techniques can include, but are not limited to, therapy sessions spent walking or sitting in nature, immersive time in wilderness, horticulture therapy or therapeutic gardening (see Chapter 10), equine or animal-assisted therapy (see Chapter 9), and adventure-based activities, such as rock climbing or ropes courses (see Chapter 7) (Jordan & Hinds, 2016). Important to all of these practices, however, is the understanding that ecotherapy is not just *using* nature in therapy. A deeper understanding of the human-nature connection and the reciprocity of the relationship is critical in ecotherapy work. Clinebell's (1996) Ecological Wellness Checkup is a comprehensive exploration of an individual's relationship with nature, essentially a "do-it-yourself tool" for those desiring an "ecological check-in" (pp. 173–176). The questionnaire asks many questions about one's experience with and feelings toward the natural world, taking stock in things one is particularly "excellent" at, "doing OK but there is definitely room for improvement," or "need strengthening." After taking the assessment, Clinebell suggests that one develop a Self-Earth Care Plan to help think through ways to provide oneself and the earth the care and support needed. He recommends a wellness plan that encompasses inreach, upreach, and outreach (Clinebell, 1996).

Recent research by Reese and Myers (2012) highlighted the need to expand on the overarching concept of wellness to include *EcoWellness*. Wellness, broadly understood, is the pursuit of good health and the choices one makes in that pursuit. Reese and Myers (2012) argued that a missing component in wellness models is "a sense of appreciation, respect for, and awe of nature that results in feelings of connectedness with the natural environment and the enhancement of holistic wellness" (p. 400). EcoWellness is multifaceted and includes several components. One such component is an individual's access to nature. Not everyone has accessibility to safe natural places—a pervasive, systemic issue that affects people disproportionately depending on their race and socio-economic status (McCormick, 2017). A person is more likely to have a healthy and strong environmental identity if they have had open and safe accessibility to nature, especially as a child. Reese and Myers (2012) also identified *transcendence* as a critical factor in EcoWellness. Transcendence is the capacity to think and stretch beyond oneself in order to have strong relationships and connect to deeper levels of understanding. To have the capacity for transcendence, spirituality and a connection to community are critical. Spirituality does not necessarily need to be in the form of a religious belief, although it can be. Spirituality could also be a deep, transcendent connection to something, such as a favorite spot by the river. Community encompasses not just people, family, ethnic groups, or neighborhoods but also the biodiverse community surrounding us.

Deeper Ecotherapy

Næss (1990) called for a deep ecology movement, one in which "human and non-human life on Earth has intrinsic value" (p. 29) but also stressing that if one ascribes to an ecological platform, one must also actively participate and implement necessary change. Buzzell (2016) also emphasized the need for deeper ecotherapy. She terms this *Level 1* and *Level 2 ecotherapies.* To Buzzell, Level 1 ecotherapy is *human-centered nature therapy,* which, simply stated, is going into nature and benefitting from its healing powers. There is evidence to suggest nature can improve one's mood and well-being in as little as five minutes (Frumkin et al., 2017). As such, Level 1 ecotherapy is beneficial in itself. Buzzell argued, however, that Level 1 ecotherapy misses a critical piece, the overarching pain and suffering currently experienced by nature and humans and its effects on the health of both. Buzzell's Level 2 ecotherapy is a "Circle of Reciprocal Healing," stating that "there can be no true human health on a sick planet" (p. 71). Level 2 ecotherapy conceptualizes healing oneself involves healing the planet. Level 2 ecotherapy involves expanding clinical work with clients to include a deeper understanding of their own connection to nature. Understanding that some anxieties may manifest in deep concern about the health of the earth may be a step in the right direction. For another, Level 2 ecotherapy brought out a deep connection and concern for the welfare of animals, especially those deemed strays or abandoned.

Level 2 ecotherapists are deliberate with their interactions with nature. If horticultural therapy (see Chapter 10) is a preferred technique, they stress the use of plants that are indigenous to their geographical location and beneficial to local wildlife. A Level 2 ecotherapist utilizing animal-assisted therapy allows the animal space and freedom to interact with human clients and never forces the interaction. A client who deeply cared for animals, especially dogs, can begin to volunteer in a no-kill shelter, gently giving the dogs the love and attention that they may need. In addition to dogs, horses can be powerful therapeutic partners. Research has suggested that horses can innately tune into human emotion, easily sensing anxiety (Hinds & Ranger, 2016). Human and horse must work together to stay grounded and relaxed if any interactions are to happen (see Chapter 9). In Level 2 animal-assisted therapy, the interaction between animal and human must be mutually beneficial. Therapists can cultivate their own practice of Level 2 ecotherapy. By tuning into the specific needs of the local ecosystem, there are many ways that therapists can incorporate Level 2 ecotherapy into their work.

Through his research, Reese (2016), a counselor educator and clinician, identified six underlying factors important for therapists wishing to include ecotherapy in their practice. First, the therapist, especially if currently working in traditional settings, must assess a client's connection to nature before introducing nature into their work together. A second important consideration is that the therapist must have a strong working knowledge of the concepts of ecotherapy and EcoWellness before doing the work with others. Third, the informed consent process must be beyond what is typical and address the purpose, benefits, and risks of working in the natural world. Fourth, when working in natural settings, protecting confidentiality can sometimes be challenging. It is important to have those conversations before going outside. Fifth, it is important to honor a client's nature worldview, not just project your own onto the client. Sixth, access to nature should be safe (Reese, 2016). These components of EcoWellness are critical to ecotherapeutic work and can be used both as a guide for conceptualization as well as a theoretical underpinning of this approach. The following case vignette provides an example of how ecotherapy, specifically reconnecting clients with their relationship with nature, can be healing.

Case Vignette

Jenna, a woman in her mid-20s, came to my practice struggling with the relationships in her life. As with all new clients, I discussed with her the tenets of my ecotherapy practice, being sure to cover ethical considerations, confidentiality, and safety. After the initial formalities, we began our journey together as counselor and client forming a new relationship, one that at its core is meant to provide solace, healing, empathy, understanding, and unconditional positive regard. Yet my work with Jenna is different, as I have a therapeutic partner with nature, adding a powerful dynamic.

Jenna and I met for our weekly sessions in one of three places. Sometimes we met in a nearby park known for its lush gardens and dedicated volunteer horticulturalists. We would stroll the grounds observing the changes in landscape, watching flowers bloom, and stopping at the koi pond to sit calmly, watching the fish slowly moving around the lily pads. Other days we met at a hiking spot, following a wooded trail, meandering through the trees. Sometimes we met at a local beach where we would sit and listen to the rolling waves, watching the sunset behind us spreading pink, blue, and purple in the sky. I allowed Jenna to pick the spot and noticed that it often matched her mood. There were days when our brisk walking matched her need to do extensive processing. Other days, we would sit and allow space for calmness and rejuvenation. The therapeutic work proceeded as would one of my typical couch sessions.

We explored her childhood, assessed the qualities of early attachments, processed significant life events, discussed her current relationship, reinforced her strengths, and strategized various coping skills.

As Jenna and I got to know each other, we explored her early childhood experiences. Jenna grew up in a small town in the outer banks of North Carolina. As such, her childhood memories were filled with hot summer days and the relief brought by jumping into the cool waves of the Atlantic Ocean. She roamed the dunes and sand drifts of the coast, finding shade from the dune grasses, and collecting shells along the water. The dunes and the beach were Jenna's special places. During her childhood, the outer banks experienced a boom in commercial development. Jenna and her family watched as streets were carved into the sand and paved over. Jenna watched stilted house after house being erected on the vast coastline, effectively cutting her off from the place she used to roam free. As we spoke of these memories, tears welled in Jenna's eyes. "Why am I crying?" she wondered aloud between deep breaths, tears streaming down her face, "I had a happy childhood. My parents loved me. I had everything I ever needed." Through our work, Jenna began to understand that the pervasive sadness of her adolescence was greatly influenced by watching her beloved coastal dunes being bulldozed and built into human fortresses. She acknowledged the grief she felt and sense of loss she experienced. Through this lens, Jenna began to explore her deep expression of caring and compassion in all of her relationships and how, sometimes, this caused pain and feelings of betrayal.

Over the time Jenna and I worked together, we covered dozens of miles. She worked through problems in her relationship, learned new coping skills to manage anxiety, let go of things beyond her control, analyzed the ways that she can make her interactions with family and friends healthier, and developed new strategies for creating boundaries. She also rekindled her deep love for the ocean. Living in New Jersey, she had access to many beaches but resonated with the ones that had open, expansive dunes, free of houses, shops, and busy boardwalks. She made time in her daily and weekly life to replenish herself at the shore. Simultaneously, she became active in a local group working to protect a stretch of land scarred by the waste of industrialized and illegal dumping. She reached out to local and state representatives, working together with an environmental group, getting the attention the site needed for environmental cleanup. She was surprised by her activism and learned she had a skill for advocacy work. She felt empowered by her own growth and also by knowing she was caring for the earth. Jenna is a true success story, but in all my years of rekindling connections with nature, even the greatest naysayer can acknowledge the healing power of her relationship with the earth and joy she found being in nature.

Conclusion

This chapter provides an overview of the historical development of ecopsychology or "psychology as if the whole earth mattered" (Roszak et al., 1995, p. 12) including a deeper understanding of the emergence of the movement. Concepts of ecogrief, biophobia, and EcoWellness were discussed. Research regarding ways that reconnecting to nature can be beneficial, especially in the context of mental health, were reviewed and the tenets of ecotherapy were discussed offering an enhanced approach to conceptualizing and healing clients. Finally, the case of Jenna was presented as an illustration of an ecotherapeutic approach to clinical mental health. This chapter provided a foundation for the additional outdoor and nature-based therapeutic approaches discussed in this book.

References

Bratman, G. N., Hamilton, J. P., Hahn, K. S., Daily, G. C., & Gross, J. J. (2015). Nature experience reduces rumination and subgenual prefrontal cortex activation. *Proceedings of the National Academy of Sciences of the United States of America, 112,* 8567–8572.

Brymer, E., Cuddihy, T. F., & Sharma-Brymer, V. (2010). The role of nature-based experiences in the development and maintenance of wellness. *Asia-Pacific Journal of Health, Sport and Physical Education, 1,* 21–27.

Buzzell, L. (2016). The many ecotherapies. In M. Jordan & J. Hinds (Eds.), *Ecotherapy: Theory, research and practice.* (pp. 70–80). London, England: Macmillan International Higher Education.

Buzzell, L. & Chalquist, C. (Eds.) (2009). *Ecotherapy: Healing with nature in mind.* San Francisco, CA: Sierra Club Books.

Carrell, S. (2018). Scottish GPs to begin prescribing rambling and birdwatching. *The Guardian,* International Edition. Retrieved December 3, 2019 from https://www.theguardian.com/uk-news/2018/oct/05/scottish-gps-nhs-begin-prescribing-rambling-birdwatching

Clinebell, H. (1996). *Ecotherapy: Healing ourselves, healing the earth.* Minneapolis, MN: Augsburg Fortress Press.

Conn, S. (1995). When the earth hurts, who responds? In T. Roszak, M. E. Gomes, & A. D. Kanner (Eds.), *Ecopsychology: Restoring the earth, healing the mind* (pp. 156–171). Berkeley, CA: The University of California Press.

Cozolino, L. (2014). *The neuroscience of human relationships* (2nd ed.). New York, NY: Norton.

Diffey, B. L. (2011). An overview analysis of the time people spend outdoors. *British Journal of Dermatology, 164*(4), 848–854.

Doherty, T. J. & Clayton, S. (2011). The psychological impacts of global climate change. *American Psychologist, 66*(4), 265–276.

Faber Taylor, A. & Kuo, F. E. (2011). Could exposure to everyday green spaces help treat ADHD? Evidence from children's play settings. *Applied Psychology: Health and Well-Being, 3,* 281–303.

Fromm, E. (1973). *The anatomy of human destructiveness*. New York, NY: Holt, Rinehart & Winston.

Frumkin, H., Bratman, G. N., Breslow, S. J., Cochran, B., Kahn, P. H., Jr., Lawler, J. J., ... Wood, S. A. (2017). Nature contact and human health: A research agenda. *Environmental Health Perspectives, 125*(7), 075001.

Hinds, J. & Ranger, L. (2016). Equine-assisted therapy: Developing theoretical context. In M. Jordan & J. Hinds (Eds.), *Ecotherapy: Theory, research and practice* (pp. 187–198). London, England: Macmillan International Higher Education.

Jordan, M. & Hinds, J. (Eds.). (2016). *Ecotherapy: Theory, research and practice*. London, England: Macmillan International Higher Education.

Jylhä, K. M. & Akrami, N. (2015). Social dominance orientation and climate change denial: The role of dominance and system justification. *Personality and Individual Differences, 86*, 108–111.

Kahn, P. H. & Hasbach, P. H. (Eds.). (2012). *Ecopsychology: Science, totems, and the technological species*. Cambridge, MA: MIT Press.

Krčmářová, J. (2009). E. O. Wilson's concept of biophilia and the environmental movement in the USA. *Klaudyán: Internet Journal of Historical Geography and Environmental History, 6*, 4–17. Retrieved November 15, 2019 from www.klaudyan.cz

Maller, C., Henderson-Wilson, C., & Townsend, M. (2009). Rediscovering nature in everyday settings: Or how to create healthy environments and healthy people. *EcoHealth, 6*, 553–556.

McCormick, R. (2017). Does access to green space impact the mental well-being of children: A systematic review. *Journal of Pediatric Nursing, 37*, 3–7.

Morrison, C. & Gore, H. (2010). Relationship between excessive internet use and depression: A questionnaire-based study of 1,319 young people and adults. *Psychopathology, 43*, 121–126.

Næss, A. (1990). *Ecology, community and lifestyle: Outline of an ecosophy*. Cambridge, England: Cambridge University Press.

Ojala, M. (2018). Eco-anxiety. *RSA Journal, 16*(4), 10–15.

Reese, R. F. (2016). EcoWellness and guiding principles for the ethical integration of nature into counseling. *International Journal for the Advancement of Counselling, 38*, 345–57.

Reese, R. F. & Myers, J. E. (2012). EcoWellness: The missing factor in holistic wellness models. *Journal of Counseling & Development, 90*(4), 400–406.

Roszak, T. (1992). *The voice of the earth*. New York, NY: Simon & Schuster.

Roszak, T., Gomes, M. E., & Kanner, A. D. (Eds.). (1995). *Ecopsychology: Restoring the earth, healing the mind*. San Francisco, CA: Sierra Club Books.

Thorp, A. A., Owen, N., Neuhaus, M., & Dunstan, D. W. (2011). Sedentary behaviors and subsequent health outcomes in adults: A systematic review of longitudinal studies, 1996–2011. *American Journal of Preventive Medicine, 41*, 207–215.

Torio, C. M., Encinosa, W., Berdahl, T., McCormick, M. C., & Simpson, L. A. (2015). Annual report on health care for children and youth in the United States: National estimates of cost, utilization and expenditures for children with mental health conditions. *Academic Pediatrics, 15*(1), 19–35.

Waller, V. (2009). Information systems 'in the wild': Supporting activity in the world. *Behavior and Information Technology, 28,* 577–688.

Wilson, E. O. (1984). *Biophilia.* Cambridge, MA: Harvard University.

White, R. & Heerwagen, J. (1998). Nature and mental health: Biophilia and biophobia. In A. Lundberg (Ed.), *The environment and mental health: A guide for clinicians* (pp. 175–192). Mahwah, NJ: Erlbaum.

Chapter 4

Psychological First Aid for Outdoor Programs

Christine Lynn Norton, Anita R. Tucker, and Scott Bandoroff

Introduction

Risk has typically been defined as a situation that exposes one to physical or psychological danger, and yet risk-taking has also been conceived of as an important component of human development, particularly for youth and young adults (Lightfoot, 1997; Steinberg, 2007). Taking risks in outdoor program settings can propel us to grow and develop in new ways by exposing us to potentially both physically and interpersonally novel environments and situations, which may help us manage our fears and anxieties (Harper, Rose, & Segal, 2019). Many of the outdoor therapies mentioned in this book rely on experiential learning (see Chapter 2), or learning by doing, and can often involve risk (Morris, 2019). As such, managing risk in outdoor settings has been an important concept, given that participants often have to manage varying environmental factors and potentially challenging activities. In this context, it becomes important to make programmatic and facilitative judgments and decisions about types and levels of risk.

In assessing the ability and behavior of our participants, we must also consider their social, emotional, and mental health and the risks associated with them. We often invite participants to engage with others in unfamiliar settings or activities, which also requires an assessment of their stress tolerance and coping capacity. Outdoor programs employ staff as facilitators, leaders, and educators and it is important to identify what levels of mental health knowledge, awareness, and skills these staff might need to keep clients physically and emotionally safe. This chapter presents opportunities for practitioners to prepare themselves to address mental health challenges among participants in outdoor program settings, and important mental health prevention and response strategies to use in practice. These strategies are generally referred to as psychological first aid, an approach developed in the early 1990s, primarily in disaster and crisis response fields (Everly Jr., McCabe, Semon, Thompson, & Links, 2014; McCabe et al., 2014). We will present an overview of developing models of training, key elements, and recommendations for best practices and further research.

History of Risk Management in Outdoor Settings

Risk management in outdoor settings has evolved to include a focus on social, emotional, and psychological risks. This is especially crucial as outdoor programming has been increasingly used for therapeutic purposes in response to the increased prevalence of mental health issues among the general population (Merikangas et al., 2010). Outdoor programs, such as the National Outdoor Leadership School (NOLS) and Outward Bound (2019), have led the outdoor field in risk management practices in the United States. These organizations have recently begun focusing more on the health and well-being of students and staff, with an emphasis on assessing the physical and psychological health of participants and staff that will either support or hinder their ability to cope with the "rigor, risks, and remoteness" of outdoor programs (NOLS, 2019). Likewise, the Association for Experiential Education (2019) has suggested risk management standards to assess psychological risk as part of their accreditation for adventure and outdoor behavioral health-care programs.

Both Outward Bound and National Outdoor Leadership School have incorporated aspects of mainstream mental health trainings for non-clinical staff such as Psychological First Aid and Mental Health First Aid, and many outdoor programs have trained their staff in the Clinical First Responder training. These trainings represent the integration of evidence-based mental health intervention skills for non-clinical staff that can be adapted for outdoor settings. These trainings focus on mental health response skills that can help staff respond effectively to mental health crises in outdoor settings.

Ethical Considerations in Psychological First Aid

According to the World Health Organization (2019), one in four people globally will be affected by mental or neurological disorders at some point in their lives. Likewise, there has been an increase in complex trauma where individuals are exposed to multiple traumas, which can affect people's self-regulation, relationship skills, and coping capacity (Kliethermes, Schacht, & Drewry, 2014; Spinazzola, 2005). Given the global prevalence of mental health disorders and trauma in the general population, we can expect to be faced with these issues in outdoor program settings. Furthermore, outdoor and environmental programs must prepare staff to try to prevent, and respond when necessary, to mental health crises in the field as these programs can increase the stress level of participants through novel environments, challenging activities, group living, and other stressors (Mutz & Müller, 2016). Psychological first aid, in this case, becomes more important, as non-clinical staff should be able to assess and monitor the risk and protective factors of both the individual participant and the group. Psychological first aid for paraprofessionals has a long-standing practice with training in place for decades for emergency and disaster relief staff and volunteers (see Everly Jr., & Lating, 2017).

Assessment of stress and resilience levels is especially important among children, youth, and young adults in outdoor programs. The added neurological and developmental vulnerabilities of this population, along with the early onset of mental health disorders, which frequently occur in adolescence, should be considered as unique factors in psychological first aid (Dahl, 2004; Heyes & Hiu, 2019). Trainers targeting programs serving young people should provide information about the developing brain, stages of psychosocial and sexual identity development, along with strengths-based perspectives on adolescence and young adulthood. Likewise, given what we are learning about the prevalence and neurobiology of adverse childhood experiences (Sacks, Murphey & Moore, 2014), outdoor program participants with a history of complex trauma, such as veterans, survivors of sexual abuse or domestic violence have additional needs that should be considered in psychological first aid. For this reason, key components in the assessment and management of risk should include learning about trauma-informed care approaches that lean away from coercive practice and move toward safety, choice, collaboration, trustworthiness, and empowerment (Harris & Fallot, 2001; Substance Abuse and Mental Health Services Administration, 2014).

Along with a focus on safety and well-being, psychological first aid skills are beneficial for outdoor program staff to have. Under pressure to provide quality treatment within budgetary constraints, it can be challenging to carve out time and resources to provide training necessary for staff to excel. Consequently, staff can feel overwhelmed, underprepared, and stressed, which can contribute to burnout or cause staff to leave the field prematurely (Kolaski & Taylor, 2019). Hence, it is important for programs to understand the current resources available to them to help support effective training for staff.

Psychological First Aid Approaches

We have identified four main psychological first aid training approaches that we believe can inform outdoor programs when thinking about how best to train their staff to handle emotionally and psychologically difficult situations with participants. Below we provide a brief overview of each model.

Mental Health First Aid provides non-clinical staff with basic skills "to reach out and provide initial help and support to someone who may be developing a mental health or substance use problem or experiencing a crisis" (National Council for Behavioral Health, 2019, para. 1). Training in Mental Health First Aid covers the prevalence, signs, and symptoms of prominent mental health disorders, and how to develop an action plan for a variety of situations.

Psychological First Aid is an evidence-informed approach to help children, adolescents, adults, and families in the immediate aftermath of disaster and terrorism (National Child Traumatic Stress Network, 2019). Similar to mental health first aid, training in psychological first aid has been adapted to enable non-clinical staff in outdoor settings to provide basic support and assistance in the face of situations that may overwhelm the individual's capacity to cope (Everly Jr., & Lating, 2017). The core actions of Psychological First Aid are designed to respond to mental health and behavioral challenges with compassion and empathy.

The *Behavioral First Responder* training is based on the work of Ewert and Davidson (2017) and addresses not only behavioral intervention strategies, such as motivational interviewing, behavioral contracts, and natural and logical consequences, but also introduces the concept of group management as a fundamental tool that can and should be used proactively to prevent behavioral and psychological crises in the field (Alpenglow Education, 2019).

The *Clinical First Responder* (2019) training, based off of the medical first responder model, was created by Dr. Scott Bandoroff, Dr. Sandy Newes, and Katie Asmus to help non-clinical staff in outdoor therapy and residential treatment settings become better equipped to prevent and respond to mental health crises that may arise. Mental health crises are likely to occur due to a lack of safety established by program staff and potentially the novelty of the environment (e.g., activities with too high an intensity or replicating conditions similar to previous trauma). During the training, staff learn to recognize a wide variety of psychological issues and how to prevent critical incidents and communicate effectively to de-escalate emotional crises if they happen. An offshoot of the Clinical First Responder training, Clinical First Aid, is a four-day certification for outdoor program staff working in non-clinical settings.

While these four models differ in length and depth, they all provide outdoor staff with general knowledge about mental health issues and theories, and what to pay attention to in their participants to recognize mental health crises. In addition, each model teaches different ways for staff to attend to the situation, assess for safety, de-escalate a situation if needed, and help participants cope with the issue. Both Behavioral First Responder and Clinical First Responder, which are longer and more in depth, also teach staff how to create a group environment that may prevent such crises from occurring.

Psychological First Aid Approaches in Outdoor Programming

Given the variety of approaches that exist, outdoor programs may find it challenging to determine which training would be best suited for their organization. The time and costs involved can be prohibitive, and programs often want a specialized training tailored to meet the unique needs of their staff and participants. In 2019, the lead author of this chapter consulted with the Student Conservation Association, an environmental organization in the United States, to create a custom training with the core components of the psychological first aid covered in this chapter. A methodical process was undertaken, including being trained in three of the four above-mentioned models, an in-depth content analysis of the curriculum and process of these trainings, and determining which mental health prevention and response strategies were essential to include. This review identified three main areas of content we believe should be included in psychological first aid training of outdoor staff.

Content #1: Mental Health Prevalence, Signs and Symptoms, and Population-Specific Factors

All of the psychological first aid approaches discussed in this chapter provide staff with information about the prevalence, definitions, and signs and symptoms of the most common mental health disorders. Content should be provided that covers depression and suicide, anxiety and panic attacks, self-harm, eating disorders, ADHD, substance abuse, psychosis, and other common diagnoses, in order to give staff a foundation of mental health knowledge before learning and practicing mental health prevention and response strategies. Likewise, given the young populations that many outdoor programs work with, the training should also provide information about the adolescent brain and stages of psychosocial development. We believe it is imperative that all mental health training for outdoor programs include population-specific information about development, risk and protective factors, and other multicultural considerations.

Content #2: Group Management Strategies for Outdoor Staff as Prevention

Beyond addressing how to respond to a crisis, the Clinical First Responder and Behavior First Responder trainings take into consideration the importance of group management, and moreover, the creation and maintenance of a physical and emotional safety and an inclusive community. Research from residential treatment has shown that group management and facilitation skills, such as those mentioned in Chapter 2, can reduce the incidence of behavioral incidents (Izzo et al., 2016). Therefore, we believe that outdoor staff would benefit from training in the following components to build and maintain a healthy group culture as a way of preventing mental health crises from happening in the first place:

- Creating group norms
- Appropriately using natural and logical consequences and behavioral contracts
- Understanding stages of group development
- Facilitating experiential community-building activities that foster social and emotional learning
- Facilitating therapeutic individual and group conversations
- Prioritizing issues of diversity, equity, and inclusion.

In addition to teaching group management skills, outdoor program staff could learn other mental health crisis prevention strategies, such as addressing the basic need of their participants (Noltemeyer, Bush, Patton, & Bergen, 2012), the effects of adverse childhood experiences (Oral et al., 2016), utilizing choice theory to better understand human behavior and motivation (Bradley, 2014), developing participants' social and emotional skills (Ashdown & Bernard, 2012), and teaching brain-based mindfulness strategies to enhance safety and judgment in the field (Ren et al., 2011). These relational tools can help create a sense of safety and belonging, which Lester and Cross (2015) have found to be strong protective factors in the face of mental health challenges.

Content #3: Crisis Intervention—Mental Health Response Strategies for Outdoor Staff

Even when intentional strategies are implemented to prevent the occurrence of mental health crises in the field, there is always the possibility that an individual's coping capacity can be overwhelmed by a precipitating event. In this case, staff must also be equipped to respond compassionately and professionally in the face of a mental health crisis. Based on the various approaches to psychological first aid, we deem the following knowledge, skills, and abilities essential for staff to be able to effectively cope with and respond to psychological and behavioral incidents in the field:

- Assessment of possible harm to self or others
  - Self-injury
  - Suicide ideation

- • Physical aggression and violence
- • Professional requirements to report harm
- De-escalation and grounding techniques
  - • Anger management
  - • Crisis intervention
  - • Co- and self-regulation
  - • Mindfulness
- Communication skills
  - • Listen, affirm, validate (Clinical First Responder, 2019)
  - • Assess, listen, give reassurance, encourage, help, and support (National Council for Behavioral Health, 2019)
- Trauma-informed practice behaviors
  - • Participant-centered
  - • Physical and emotional safety
  - • Psychological first aid when necessary

These are a few key areas in which staff in outdoor program settings can be trained to assist with psychological risk in the field and respond effectively to a crisis. Along with training content, it is important to consider the process by which this vital information will be delivered. All of the approaches mentioned in this chapter incorporate experiential and interactive activities in teaching mental health prevention and response skills. Providing experiential learning and hands-on opportunities can help outdoor program staff to process information and reflect upon real-life applications. This, we feel, is key to learning the skills needed to navigate these experiences (Sand, Elison-Bowers, Wing, & Kendrick, 2014). It should be noted that online virtual learning activities are becoming more engaging as technology improves, and there are ways for people to practice their skills in this setting as well. What follows is a case example of an outdoor program staff member responding effectively to a mental health crisis which illustrates the three areas of content shared above.

Case Vignette

Joey was a 16-year-old male student on a 28-day expedition backpacking course through a wilderness leadership school. Young participants, like Joey, elected to attend the course, and no clinicians were involved in any aspect of the program. The outdoor staff utilized wilderness activities, group process, and skill-based instruction to help students work on leadership skills, such as communication, conflict resolution, coping skills, and self-esteem. Students often came on the course who were struggling to find a sense of direction and were interested in an experience outside of school.

Joey expressed feeling as though this was not the right setting for him, upon arriving to the course. He expressed hopelessness about whether he would be able to adjust to the new outdoor setting. However, after Joey started getting to know his group, he began to settle in quite well. His group was physically and emotionally safe, and overall high functioning as observed by staff. They supported one another, had fun, and were practicing both the expedition skills and leadership skills with each other consistently. The group became committed to goals that could help with life at home, such as improving their schoolwork.

In the early part of the course, Joey expressed negative thought patterns portraying low self-esteem. For example, when too many instructions were given to him at once, Joey would sometimes shut down and take space for himself away from the group. Overall, however, these moments were few and far between. When they did occur, Joey and staff were able to negotiate for him to take some private space and could help to regulate his emotional state, before returning to the group. Joey was quite self-aware and could discuss his thoughts and feelings openly.

Toward the end of the 28-day expedition, a peer was facilitating a group learning activity focused on trust. In the initiative, one of Joey's peers was directed to intentionally break the trust of the group in a small way. The experiential component of the lesson was designed intentionally to show how hard it can be to build trust, and yet how easily it can be broken. The staff had facilitated this lesson many times, and it often resonated with the participants experiences at home. Yet, in all of the times it was previously facilitated, the students recognized the 'breaking trust' behavior was part of a lesson, and did not take it too seriously.

Unexpectedly, when the peer simulated breaking trust with her team, Joey reacted explosively. He stood up and yelled angrily at the peer: "Why would you do that? You are so mean! I can't believe you would do this to us!" The group was stunned. They had not seen this type of behavior from Joey before. An instructor intervened to explain that the student had been asked to take this action as a part of the lesson, but before the instructor could get a few words out, Joey began angrily yelling at her: "This place is awful. I can't be here. I can't believe you would treat people like this." As he further escalated, he began throwing sticks and rocks in the vicinity of the group, while not aiming at any of his peers. The instructor had the group move further up the hill to give for their safety and to provide Joey with some space. The instructor provided some distance between herself and Joey and calmly stated, "Joey, I can see you are having a hard time right now. It is ok if you want to throw sticks and rocks so long as they are not directed at anyone."

Joey continued to throw things, while speaking, mainly to himself, about the precipitating situation. The instructor remained in proximity while allowing Joey to de-escalate. After about ten minutes, Joey collapsed on the ground and began sobbing. The instructor reminded him that she was there for him if he wanted to talk or needed anything.

After a few minutes, Joey began talking to the nearby instructor. He expressed embarrassment and shame at his reaction, though stood steadfast in his belief that the lesson was not fair, and his peer should not have acted in that way. His thoughts continued to represent hopelessness and low self-esteem which had come out at other moments previously during the expedition. However, as Joey continued to converse with the instructor, his thinking became increasingly more focused on the present moment, rather than the previous situation which had sparked the situation.

The instructor made sure that Joey felt safe. They worked together to create a plan for how he would return to the group. After such an outburst, the instructor recognized that other students may be scared or worried, so a plan was made for him to provide some information to the other students about what had occurred, while maintaining the level of privacy that he needed for the more personal aspects of the story. They agreed to check in later that day to assess how he was doing after some time removed from the situation. They also discussed a plan for if a similar reaction occurred again in the future. The instructor also highlighted some of the positive aspects of the situation. For example, Joey was not aggressive toward another person. He managed to remove himself from the group and de-escalate. The two also explored what other coping skills might be helpful in the future.

As a result of the training the outdoor staff had in psychological first aid, they were able to recognize how a student could be triggered by a scenario that had not triggered students in this situation previously. They acted non-judgmentally in reaction to his outburst and provided a safe space for him to release his anger, while also keeping the other students safe. The outdoor staff reported the incident to their superiors, understanding they were not trained at a level to determine someone's mental health status beyond what the student self-reported. They also understood the importance of the group in this process, and how critical a restorative process is after a situation like this occurs within a group in order to ensure a sense of safety for all participants, including Joey. The training in psychological first aid could have played a role in facilitating a positive outcome for the individual and the group in this situation.

Conclusion

The outdoor program staff in this case vignette were given effective training in psychological first aid and were therefore able to respond calmly and compassionately to a participant in crisis, while at the same time, maintain care for the group. Having an existing knowledge of mental health signs and symptoms, along with crisis prevention and response skills, allowed the instructor to respond in a way that de-escalated the student's behavior. The instructor was able to create and maintain a physically and emotionally safe environment in the face of a client crisis, by listening empathetically to the participant and behavior contracting.

We believe that training and practices in outdoor programming need to reflect the prevalence of trauma and mental health disorders among the general population. There is a need for non-clinical staff to gain more training in how to prevent and respond to mental health issues in outdoor settings (Ewert & Davidson, 2017). Although we are not suggesting that all staff in outdoor programs need to participate in specialized training, we do believe that outdoor staff would benefit from learning these skills to help respond to mental health issues that may arise in the field.

References

Alpenglow Education. (2019). Behavioral first responder certification. Retrieved August 23, 2010 from https://www.alpengloweducation.com/bfr

Ashdown, D. M. & Bernard, M. E. (2012). Can explicit instruction in social and emotional learning skills benefit the social-emotional development, well-being, and academic achievement of young children? *Early Childhood Education Journal, 39*(6), 397–405.

Association for Experiential Education. (2019). Accreditation for adventure and outdoor behavioral healthcare programs. Retrieved August 24, 2019 from https://www.aee.org/accreditations

Bradley, E. L. (2014). Choice theory and reality therapy: An overview. *International Journal of Choice Theory and Reality Therapy, 34*(1), 6–14.

Clinical First Responder. (2019). Clinical First Responder training & testimonials. Retrieved January 19, 2020 from https://peakexperiencetraining.com/clinical-first-responder/

Dahl, R. E. (2004). Adolescent brain development: A period of vulnerabilities and opportunities. Keynote address. *Annals of the New York Academy of Sciences, 1021*(1), 1–22.

Everly, G. S. Jr., McCabe, O. L., Semon, N. L., Thompson, C. B., & Links, J. M. (2014). The development of a model of psychological first aid for non-mental health trained public health personnel: The Johns Hopkins RAPID-PFA. *Journal of Public Health Management and Practice, 20*, S24–S29.

Everly, G. S. Jr., & Lating, J. M. (2017). *The Johns Hopkins guide to psychological first aid*. Baltimore, MA: JHU Press.

Ewert, A. & Davidson, C. (2017). *Behavior and group management in outdoor adventure education: Theory, research and practice*. New York, NY: Routledge.

Harper, N. J., Rose, K., & Segal, D. (2019). *Nature-based therapy: A practitioner's guide to working outdoors with children, youth, and families*. Gabriola Island, Canada: New Society Publishers.

Harris, M. & Fallot, R. D. (Eds.). (2001). *Using trauma theory to design service systems: New directions for mental health services*. San Francisco, CA: Jossey-Bass.

Heyes, S. B. & Hiu, C. F. (2019). The adolescent brain: Vulnerability and opportunity. UNICEF: Office of Research-Innocenti. Retrieved August 24, 2019 from https://www.unicef-irc.org/article/1149-the-adolescent-brain-vulnerability-and-opportunity.html

Izzo, C. V., Smith, E. G., Holden, M. J., Norton, C. I., Nunno, M. A., & Sellers, D. E. (2016). Intervening at the setting level to prevent behavioral incidents in residential child care: Efficacy of the CARE program model. *Prevention Science*, 17(5), 554–564.

Kliethermes, M., Schacht, M., & Drewry, K. (2014). Complex trauma. *Child and Adolescent Psychiatric Clinics*, 23(2), 339–361.

Kolaski, A. Z. & Taylor, J. M. (2019). Critical factors for field staff: The relationship between burnout, coping, and vocational purpose. *Journal of Experiential Education*. Advanced online publication.

Lester, L. & Cross, D. (2015). The relationship between school climate and mental and emotional wellbeing over the transition from primary to secondary school. *Psychology of Well-Being*, 5(1), 9.

Lightfoot, C. (1997). *The culture of adolescent risk-taking*. New York, NY: The Guilford Press.

Merikangas, K. R., He, J. P., Burstein, M., Swanson, S. A., Avenevoli, S., Cui, L., …, & Swendsen, J. (2010). Lifetime prevalence of mental disorders in US adolescents: Results from the National Comorbidity Survey Replication–Adolescent Supplement (NCS-A). *Journal of the American Academy of Child & Adolescent Psychiatry*, 49(10), 980–989.

McCabe, O. L., Everly, G. S. Jr., Brown, L. M., Wendelboe, A. M., Abd Hamid, N. H., Tallchief, V. L., & Links, J. M. (2014). Psychological first aid: A consensus-derived, empirically supported, competency-based training model. *American Journal of Public Health*, 104(4), 621–628.

Morris, T. H. (2019). Experiential learning–A systematic review and revision of Kolb's model. *Interactive Learning Environments*, 1–14. doi:10.1080/10494 820.2019.1570279

Mutz, M. & Müller, J. (2016). Mental health benefits of outdoor adventures: Results from two pilot studies. *Journal of Adolescence*, 49, 105–114.

National Child Traumatic Stress Network. (2019). About PFA. Retrieved August 30, 2019 from https://www.nctsn.org/treatments-and-practices/psychological-first-aid-and-skills-for-psychological-recovery/about-pfa

National Council for Behavioral Health. (2019). Mental health first aid: What you learn. Retrieved August 24, 2019 from https://www.mentalhealthfirstaid.org/take-a-course/what-you-learn/

National Outdoor Leadership School. (2019). Risk management at NOLS. Retrieved August 24, 2019 from https://www.nols.edu/media/filer_public/14/82/148290c5-a3ed-40d1-b289-4a9b2a39429b/risk-management-at-nols-2019.pdf

Noltemeyer, A., Bush, K., Patton, J., & Bergen, D. (2012). The relationship among deficiency needs and growth needs: An empirical investigation of Maslow's theory. *Children and Youth Services Review*, 34(9), 1862–1867.

Oral, R., Ramirez, M., Coohey, C., Nakada, S., Walz, A., Kuntz, A., ..., Peek-Asa, C. (2016). Adverse childhood experiences and trauma informed care: The future of healthcare. *Pediatric Research*, *79*(1–2), 227–233.

Outward Bound. (2019). Safety and risk management. Retrieved on August 24, 2019 from https://www.outwardbound.org/about-outward-bound/outward-bound-today/safety/

Ren, J., Huang, Z., Luo, J., Wei, G., Ying, X., Ding, Z., & Luo, F. (2011). Meditation promotes insightful problem-solving by keeping people in a mindful and alert conscious state. *Science China Life Sciences*, *54*(10), 961–965.

Sacks, V., Murphey, D., & Moore, K. (2014). *Adverse childhood experiences: National and state-level prevalence*. Washington, DC: Center for Victim Research.

Sand, J. N., Elison-Bowers, P., Wing, T. J., & Kendrick, L. (2014). Experiential learning and clinical education. *Academic Exchange Quarterly*, *18*(4), 43–48.

Spinazzola, J. (2005). National survey on complex trauma exposure, outcome, and intervention among children and adolescents. *Psychiatric Annals*, *35*(8), 624–624.

Steinberg, L. (2007). Risk taking in adolescence: New perspectives from brain and behavioral science. *Current Directions in Psychological Science*, *16*(2), 55–59.

Student Conservation Association. (2019). About. Retrieved August 30, 2019 from https://www.thesca.org/about

Substance Abuse and Mental Health Services Administration. (2014). *Concept of trauma and guidance for a trauma-informed care approach*. U.S. Department of Health and Human Services.

World Health Organization. (2019). World health report. Retrieved August 24, 2019 from https://www.who.int/whr/2001/media_centre/press_release/en

Chapter 5

Indigenous Land-Based Healing Pedagogies

From the Ground Up

Nicholas XEMŦOLTW̱ Claxton

ŁE, ȻÁNEK̲ TŦE TEṈEW̱ (The land is the healer).
~SENĆOŦEN expression

Introduction

Indigenous peoples in Canada, and around the world, had societies that developed and evolved over thousands and thousands of years—however, many, if not all Indigenous people's oral histories state that they have been present on their homelands since the time of creation. Each Indigenous nation has an intricate society founded upon their unique Indigenous knowledge, contained in their language, infused with their worldview, and rooted in their land. Their knowledge system is a unique way of living and being in the world, and ways of relating to each other, and to the land. For Indigenous nations, the land is vital, the land is everything (Alfred, 2017). The truth is, Indigenous nations have never been conquered, or otherwise sold, ceded, or given away their lands or nationhood, and continue to adhere to their own forms of sovereignty and nationhood (Claxton & Price, 2020). There is a growing movement of Indigenous resurgence within and by Indigenous communities in an effort to re-establish, revitalize, and strengthen Indigenous connections to land (Simpson, 2014), and these methodologies, emerging from Indigenous knowledges and paradigms, are diverse and specific to Indigenous peoples and their lands (Tuck & McKenzie, 2015). This chapter is an example of Indigenous resurgence through land-based healing in W̱SÁNEĆ territories that builds on work being done within education (Claxton & Rodriguez de France, 2019) and carries with it a long-term vision and focus for Indigenous children and youth.

Colonization in Canada has attempted to dispossess Indigenous nations and peoples from their lands and had detrimental effects on Indigenous relationships to land (Tuck & Yang, 2012). Many Indigenous worldviews, as with Indigenous languages, are threatened in Canada (First Peoples' Cultural Council, 2018). Fostering Indigenous resurgence in Indigenous children and youth is to create learning and teaching opportunities where they can grow up intimately related to and strongly connected to their homelands, immersed in their languages and spiritual worldviews, and practicing and embodying their cultural practices and traditions. The land is the teacher and also the healer (Meyer, 2008). The phrase "ŁE, ȻÁNEK̲ TᵻE TENEW̲" expresses this concept in SENĆOŦEN (the language of the W̲SÁNEĆ People), which translates into "the land is the healer."

Settler colonialism, through the implementation of the Indian Act (in Canada) and the reserve system, and state-run education and schooling have only served to sever Indigenous peoples from their lands and attempt to assimilate them into the mainstream, disrupting this healing relationship (Morgensen, 2011). It is very important to explore the development of land-based pedagogies *from the ground up*. In this chapter, I share a W̲SÁNEĆ perspective that will foster the connection of W̲SÁNEĆ youth to their homelands and strengthen their identities as W̲SÁNEĆ people, through language, story, and connection to place. This land-based pedagogy is also valuable for Indigenous peoples from other nations, as it provides a window of common understanding to share and relate to the depth of Indigenous connections to land. Lavallee and Poole (2010) suggested that health and healing for Indigenous people cannot occur without recognition of the harm that has come from colonization. Land-based pedagogy is also valuable for non-Indigenous peoples to provide an opportunity to foster and create a depth of understanding, acknowledgement, and respect for Indigenous ways of being. This can hopefully lead the way to meaningful reconciliation in alignment with the Truth and Reconciliation Commission of Canada's Calls to Action (2015) and the United Nations Declaration on the Rights of Indigenous Peoples (United Nations, 2007). These documents provide a framework for all levels of government, the corporate and not-for-profit sectors, and Canadian society as a whole to take specific actions to redress the negative consequences and legacy of colonization in general, and the harms suffered due to the residential school system specifically (Regan, 2010). With the aim of reconciliation between Canadians and Indigenous peoples, and relative to Indigenous land-based pedagogy, the calls to action include, for example, the development of culturally appropriate curricula, acknowledgement of language rights, and to ensure self-determination in spiritual matters, ritual, and celebration.

This chapter is about sharing my land-based healing pedagogy (i.e. method of teaching) that is rooted in my learning, or perhaps 'unlearning' and 're-learning,' rooted in the Indigenous knowledge of the W̲SÁNEĆ homelands and peoples. Indigenous knowledges are diverse and represent a diversity of ways of understanding the world. Indigenous peoples and knowledge systems have developed from generations of being in relationships with, living with, and depending on the physical and spiritual worlds, most importantly, being on the land. Therapeutic practice with Indigenous peoples is incomplete without Indigenous knowledge and access to, and intimate relationship with the land. For clarity, I speak of 'land' as inclusive of all elements of our homelands (water, air, forest, mountains, plant, and animal life, etc.).

Over the last number of years, I have worked in partnership with the ŁÁU, WEL, NEW Tribal School, and teach Indigenous land- and language-based courses at the University of Victoria and Camosun College here in the WSÁNEĆ territory. I have developed this pedagogy to create learning experiences grounded in the student's homelands and involve connecting those learning experiences with knowledge keepers and Indigenous knowledge systems. The pedagogy was designed to create learning experiences for Indigenous students, where they can envision their future work, as educators, child and youth care practitioners, or counselors that foster a new generation of Indigenous people who are strongly connected to their ancestral knowledge systems. This pedagogy has also been transformational for non-Indigenous students as well. For the future of our Indigenous nations, it is vital that students think and live within their Indigenous philosophies, laws, and beliefs to counter the ongoing colonialism that Indigenous nations still face today. Indigenous land-based pedagogies are vital to this. The land is our foundation, and we know that Indigenous community health and success is dependent on it (Chandler & Lalonde, 1998). When we are engaged in healing the land, we are healing ourselves.

Land-Based Healing and Indigenous Resurgence

It cannot be overstated that Indigenous societies, worldviews, and spirituality are ancient and are firmly rooted in our languages and our lands (Greenwood & Leeuw, 2007; Iseke, 2013; Simpson, 2004). Indigenous cultures in Canada, though they may be similar, are also very diverse. British Columbia, for example, is home to 60% of First Nations' languages in Canada with 32 languages and about 59 dialects (First Peoples' Cultural Council, 2018). This is to say, there is a diversity of Indigenous nations in British Columbia, though all of these nations would have similar worldviews. Each of these nations would have an ancient connection to their homelands, and each constitute nations, with their own land base. Each of these nations also share in a common experience of contact and colonization by Europeans, the displacement of knowledge and ways of knowing and the imposition of western/mainstream knowledge systems, and ways of knowing and being. These losses started with the imposition of the Indian Act and were maintained through the reserve system, residential school system, and other policies, many that continue to this day (Regan, 2010; Simpson, 2004).

There has always been a resistance by Indigenous peoples to European colonization. Children and youth have always been a beacon of hope for the future for the perpetuation of Indigenous language and culture by Indigenous nations and Indigenous leaders. For example, in 1972, the Chiefs of the National Indian Brotherhood adopted the first written policy on Indian education, entitled Indian Control of Indian Education. It was presented to Minister Jean Chretien, of Indian Affairs and Northern Development, on December 21, 1972. This policy was written as a comprehensive position paper that articulated principles of local control, parental responsibility, and culturally based curriculum. "We want education to provide the setting in which our children can develop the fundamental attitudes and values which have an honored place in Indian tradition and culture" (National Indian Brotherhood, 1972, n.p.). It was clear that Indigenous communities in Canada wanted to take a leading role in the education of their children. While the focus of the "Indian Control of Indian Education" policy paper was education, it also embodies and encompasses all aspects of the lives of children and youth, and it is entirely relevant for many working in human service fields.

Indigenous Scholarship

There is a growing movement in Indigenous scholarship and research methodologies. The scholarship that is beginning to emerge in this field is demonstrating courage and innovation and is driven by the idea that we should envision the kind methodologies and pedagogies that will foster a healthier way of life for Indigenous children and youth. Essentially, an Indigenous methodology and practice that is rooted in our languages and our lands.

There is an expanding base of research in Canada regarding the education of First Nation, Inuit, and Métis children and youth (Battiste & Barman, 1995). Non-aboriginal people have conducted much of the research, and the message is generally the same: Indigenous peoples in Canada are not succeeding in the provincial education systems. In 2006, it was reported that the rate of First Nation youth living on reserves without a high school diploma was four times higher than their non-Aboriginal counterparts in Canada (Statistics Canada, 2006). Developing educational practices about, and on the land, has shown promise for Indigenizing education (Guilar & Swallow, 2008) and health (Ritchie et al., 2015). Guilar and Swallow (2008) described:

> Bringing together people in traditionally meaningful places allows stories to be told, questions to be asked and perspectives on what learning from place can mean … Learning from place is a context for engaging in meaningful experiences and encouraging a common dialogue to explore how we can learn from our homeland. (p. 9)

As they suggested, learning from place is meaningful and transformational in education. My argument is not only about finding ways for Indigenous peoples to succeed academically in the education system, but rather, it is focused on a more deeply rooted problem, that is developing a pedagogy that both heals our nations, our lands, and our relationships. When we engage with the land and instill our ancestral languages, worldviews, epistemologies, paradigms, philosophies, and teachings in youth, this embodies what Indigenous resurgence means.

Indigenous land-based healing as Indigenous resurgence is necessarily and inherently rooted in the Land (Iseke-Barnes, 2008; Tuck & Yang, 2012). When engaging with Indigenous land-based healing, it is imperative to acknowledge, respect, include, and adhere to the relationships and connections of the local Indigenous peoples to their lands. The reconnection of the lands to the original peoples and knowledge of those lands is the significance of this pedagogy. While all lands are sacred, Indigenous communities and nations will always have a number of culturally significant places, like certain mountains, rivers, or village sites. There will also be land-based stories, language, and meaning that is connected to those places. All life, such as the plants, animals, and inanimates which occur naturally in those locations, could also have cultural and spiritual significance. When the land, life, people, story, and spirituality are reconnected and restored in the way that it was intended and gifted by the creator, that is land-based healing for Indigenous resurgence.

Healing as Land-Based Indigenous Resurgence

This project is firmly situated in and guided by the principles of Indigenous resurgence. According to Jeff Corntassel (2012), Indigenous resurgence "means having the courage and imagination to envision life beyond the state" and to "confront existing colonial institutions, structures, and policies that attempt to displace us from our homelands and relationships, which impact the health and well-being of present generations of Indigenous youth and families" (p. 89). Taiaiake Alfred (2009) suggested the process of Indigenous resurgence involves a collective community effort to achieve the following:

- The restoration of Indigenous presence(s) on the land and the revitalization of land-based practices
- An increased reliance on traditional diet(s) among Indigenous people
- The transmission of Indigenous culture, spiritual teachings, and knowledge of the land between Elders and youth
- The strengthening of familial activities and re-emergence of Indigenous cultural and social institutions as governing authorities within First Nations

- Short- and long-term initiatives and improvements in sustainable land-based economies as the primary economies of reserve-based First Nations communities and as supplemental economies for urban Indigenous communities. (p. 56)

Further to this, Leanne Betasamosake Simpson (2004) centered "Indigenous knowledge as critical" and outlines four key points for Indigenous resurgence (p. 75):

- Confront 'funding' mentality—It is time to admit that colonizing governments and private corporations are not going to fund our decolonization.
- Confronting linguistic genocide—There is little recognition or glory attached to language but without it, we will lose ourselves.
- Visioning resurgence—The importance of visioning and dreaming a better future based on our own Indigenous traditions cannot be underestimated.
- The need to awaken ancient treaty and diplomatic mechanisms— Renewing our pre-colonial treaty relationships with contemporary neighboring Indigenous nations.

As a resurgence activity in W̱SÁNEĆ territories, land-based healing was defined by Taiaiake Alfred and Leanne Simpson as the guiding framework for this community and land-based resurgence effort. My land-based healing pedagogy re-centers authentic Indigenous place and land-based knowledge, to help to instill local Indigenous worldviews and perspectives, particularly in the learning and teaching with local Indigenous children and youth.

Indigenous Resurgence

I conceptualize Indigenous resurgence in my work as a continuum from broadly understood mainstream or Western (non-Indigenous) knowledge and worldviews through to authentic Indigenous land-based knowledges, worldviews, and perspectives. It is again important to acknowledge that Indigenous knowledges and worldviews are diverse. The center of the continuum is an interface between Western and Indigenous worldviews, and that this space is also broad in scope. In this interface you would find residential schools, public schools, and band schools (funded by federal government and run by Indigenous nations). You could also identify Indigenization efforts at universities in this middle space as well (Louie, Poitras-Pratt, Hanson, & Ottmann, 2017). Indigenous resurgence moves us toward restoring authentic Indigenous land-based knowledges. This resurgence is an act of healing Indigenous communities and nations through restoring Indigenous relationships to land.

Land-Based Healing and Resurgence in W̱SÁNEĆ Territories: A Visit to ȽÁU, WEL, NEW̱

When I engage in land-based learning and teaching, I take students to culturally significant locations in W̱SÁNEĆ territories. These visits include children and youth from our W̱SÁNEĆ communities, but also with Indigenous students from other communities and nations and non-Indigenous students as well. When we are at culturally and spiritually significant places, sharing the stories that come from those places can be especially impactful. You can hear, feel, smell, touch, see, and fully experience the stories. Often, land-based stories are misunderstood to be legends or myths, that is made-up and make-believe, but in reality, they are the truths of the W̱SÁNEĆ people. When you are on the land, the stories take on a deeper meaning, and embody the truth. These land-based stories take on considerable depth in meaning. One of the most culturally important and significant places in W̱SÁNEĆ territory is ȽÁU, WEL, NEW̱ (also known as Mount Newton). The following is an important story, which connects to ȽÁU, WEL, NEW̱:

ȽÁU, WEL, NEW̱ means place of refuge, or place of escape, and is the W̱SÁNEĆ name of what people commonly known today as John Dean park at Mt. Newton. It is a sacred place of refuge for the W̱SÁNEĆ people of today and has been that since time immemorial. The mountain was named ȽÁU, WEL, NEW̱ after the great flood that had come to the land a long, long time ago. It is said that the people lived in a good way for a long time, that they lived in harmony with the land, and thus, followed the sacred teachings of XÁLS (the sacred creator). Many generations had passed and people began to forget the sacred teachings, and hence, began to live out of balance with nature. Messages came to holy people of the land that a great time of purification was coming in the form of a flood and that they should prepare themselves. The waters rose until the only land that remained was the mountain peaks. It is said that the people who forgot the sacred teachings had perished aboard their canoes, having either capsized or drifted away—never to be seen again. The people who remained tied their canoes to an arbutus tree atop a mountain. For a long time, the people remained at the mercy of the elements. And so, they prayed and prayed for mercy until one day a crow landed on the bow of one of their canoe's carrying a stick in its mouth. The people understood this to be a message that the flood was coming to an end. A mountain appeared in the distance, to which one of the people shouted in excitement, "NI QENET TŦE W̱SÁNEĆ LO, TE ȻȽ TÁȽ" (look what is emerging off in the distance, the waters are receding). Hence, the waters receded, but the people remained on the mountain that had saved them, and they discussed the sacred time that they had survived. They gave thanks to the sacred arbutus tree, vowing to never burn it. They coiled the sacred rope that had saved them and gave thanks to it as well. Then, the people gave thanks to the sacred mountain that had saved them and acknowledged it with the name ȽÁU, WEL, N̲EW̲, so that the people would never forget that sacred time and the sacred teachings carried by their ancestors. Also, the people named themselves and the land in memory of that sacred time as the emerging land, and the emerging people—W̱SÁNEĆ.

This story describes the deep history and connection of the W̱SÁNEĆ people to this place. The name of the sacred mountain and the name of the people are the same. This story is sacred and describes the deep connection to the land, and to the creator, and to creation itself. The story also describes the ability to see a sacred coiled rope (if one is of clean mind and spirit, and deeply connected to this place). From this location, you can physically see the vast majority of W̱SÁNEĆ territory. Experiencing this location and experiencing this history instills a strong sense of identity and connection to the land, and to being a W̱SÁNEĆ person. For Indigenous students from other communities/nations, this can provide an example of the depth of connection of Indigenous knowledges and languages to the land, and it inspires them to explore their connections to their own identities and homelands. For non-Indigenous peoples and students, learning from the land in this way—from Indigenous knowledge keepers of that land—that can foster a deeper sense of awareness and respect, for the peoples, and for the land. This also moves us toward reconciliation.

Another powerful story that connects to our local lands is the ṮEṮÁĆES story is as follows:

ṮEṮÁĆES is the W̱SÁNEĆ name for island, or islands. Roughly translated, it means relatives of the deep, which refers to the story of how the islands came to be. It is said that long ago XÁLS (the creator) came to W̱SÁNEĆ to change many things about the world. He came to the territory aboard a canoe at the area known to the W̱SÁNEĆ peoples as ṮIX̱EN (Cordova Spit at Saanichton Bay). XÁLS came ashore. He then walked toward the west side of the point, where he cast a black stone into the horizon, followed by another black stone, which became ȽÁUWELN̲EW̱ (Mt. Newton). XÁLS had with him a basket that he loaded with more black stones. He then walked toward ȽÁUWELN̲EW̱. Several people had witnessed the sacred spectacle, and in their curiosity, followed XÁLS to the mountain. Atop the mountain XÁLS proceeded to cast more black stones, which then made the mountains. When he ran out of stones, he turned toward the people who had followed him to the mountain and began to grab the people who were of the greatest virtue. He cast them out into the ocean and told each of them, "QEN, T TŦEN SĆÁLEĆE" (look after your relatives). They then rooted themselves deep into the ocean, becoming the islands. He was done casting people to the water and turned to those who had remained with him on the mountain and told them, "I, QEN, T SE SW̱ TȾEN SĆÁLEĆE" (And you will look after your relatives), and gestured to the ṮEṮÁĆES (islands).

This story is significant because my students can stand in the location where this happened, near the summit of ȽÁU, WEL, ṈEW, where the creator also stood. The students can also look out and view the islands from afar, the islands that were created from the ancestors of the W̱SÁNEĆ peoples. This story instills a strong sense of W̱SÁNEĆ identity, and an in-depth feeling of connection to the territory. The listener and learner develop an understanding of the extent of the W̱SÁNEĆ homelands while also have a bodily felt experience of being in that place. For W̱SÁNEĆ children and youth, this knowledge is invaluable as it is culturally grounded and learned experientially from their own people. For non-Indigenous peoples, similarly to the previous story, awareness and respect for the people and the land are fostered through learning of this story and their physical presence in the place where it is told.

While visiting this location, there is also an opportunity to learn about local ethnobotanical knowledge, or the relationship between plants and people. Local W̱SÁNEĆ knowledge of plants is profound, and as you learn about, it exemplifies the strength of the relationship to the territory, and through language. The W̱SÁNEĆ people used just about every native plant for one use or another. Plants could be used for technology, food, medicine, or as an indicator for something else. There has been significant research and documentation of the use of traditional ethnobotany of the W̱SÁNEĆ people (see Turner & Hebda, 2012; Turner, Lepofsky, & Deur, 2013).

The opportunity for learning and teaching through Indigenous land-based healing and resurgence is wide-ranging and will be specific to local peoples and their territories. Children, youth, and learners of all ages can connect with local Indigenous knowledge keepers and engage in learning from the land. This is healing. This is Indigenous resurgence.

Where Do We Go From Here?

In Canada, Indigenous peoples have been living on and together with their lands for thousands of years. Non-Indigenous and mainstream methods and approaches to education and healing could be guided by the depth of Indigenous connections to land. From the perspective of the W̱SÁNEĆ people, we have been here since the beginning, and it is the creator, XÁLS, who put us here. It is only with our presence here that a very deep and connected worldview and philosophy has developed. Western ways of knowing and being, and ways of learning and teaching, have misunderstood this.

It must be recognized that 'land based pedagogies' and 'healing practices' are enterprises that are inherently philosophical at their core. When engaging in land-based pedagogies, it is imperative to be aware of this, and to privilege and re-center local Indigenous knowledges and languages (Greenwood & Leeuw, 2007).

Despite all of their diversities, Indigenous philosophies have one thing in common; a deep seeded and spiritual connection to the land (Baskin, 2016). The environment and all living things were important to and inseparable from Indigenous worldviews. Indigenous peoples related to the land and were a part of a dynamic living system. The land was not something to be controlled, and transformed (destroyed) for monetary capital gain, it was something to be respected, as all living beings are. The connection to the environment was deep and meaningful. Our W̱SÁNEĆ elder and advisor John Elliott Sr. stated, "We have been here for a long time. During that time, we lived with the sea songs, the elements, and the lands. Our ancestors continue to teach us through our ancient language and through our presence here" (Personal communication, 2013). It is clear that language, songs, ceremony, and the land (ecosystem) are intertwined and inseparable and have been in place for millennia. It is important for health and well-being that these practices be remembered, revitalized, and carried on into the future generations (Chandler & Lalonde, 1998). We as a people have a responsibility to maintain our history and practices, for each other, and for the environment. These actions contribute to a global socio-ecological resistance to colonial structures and systems, and can promote human and environmental justice (Williams, Bunda, Claxton, & MacKinnon, 2018).

The environment, the land, and all living things are important, and more than that, integral to an Indigenous worldview. What is evident in the language, songs, ceremonies, and practices is the importance of both the physical and spiritual realms, and how they were interconnected rather than separated. Umeek, also known as Dr. Richard Atleo (2007), in his book *Tsawalk: A Nuu-chah-nulth Worldview* developed what he calls an Indigenous theory on the Nuu-chah-nuulth Nation's concept of 'heshook-ish tsawalk.' Umeek translated this to mean "everything is one." This is the Nuu-chah-nulth perspective that reality is inclusive of both the physical and the metaphysical. The spiritual world and physical world are not separate to the Nuu-chah-nulth. Similarly, our elder John Elliott Sr. said "a whole new reality is created when you connect to the spiritual world" (Personal communication, 2013). Indigenous knowledge systems and connections to land are central to the health of the land and health of our relationships to the natural world. Indigenous land-based healing can heal the land, and our connections and relationships to it. It can also benefit all people, not just Indigenous peoples.

References

Alfred, T. (2009). Colonialism and state dependency. *Journal of Aboriginal Health*, *5*(1), 42–60.

Alfred, T. (2017). It's all about the land. In P. McFarlane & N. Schabus (Eds.), *Whose land is it anyway? A manual for decolonization* (pp. 10–13). Vancouver, Canada: Federation of Post-Secondary Educators of BC.

Atleo, E. R. (2007). *Tsawalk: A Nuu-chah-nulth worldview*. Vancouver, Canada: UBC Press.

Baskin, C. (2016). Spirituality: The core of healing and social justice from an indigenous perspective. *New Directions for Adult and Continuing Education*, *152*, 51–60.

Battiste, M. & Barman, J. (1995). *First Nations education in Canada: The circle unfolds*. Vancouver, Canada: UBC Press.

Chandler, M. J. & Lalonde, C. (1998). Cultural continuity as a hedge against suicide in Canada's First Nations. *Transcultural Psychiatry*, *35*(2), 191–219.

Claxton, N. & Price, J. (2020). Whose land is it? Rethinking sovereignty in British Columbia. *BC Studies: The British Columbian Quarterly*, *204*, 115138.

Claxton, N. & Rodriguez de France, C. (2019). With roots in water: Revitalizing Straits Salish reef net fishing as education for well-being and sustainability. In L. T. Smith, E. Tuck, & K. W. Yang (Eds.), *Indigenous and decolonizing studies in education: Mapping the long view* (pp. 215–223). New York, NY: Routledge.

Corntassel, J. (2012). Re-envisioning resurgence: Indigenous pathways to decolonization and sustainable self-determination. *Decolonization: Indigeneity, Education & Society*, *1*(1), 86–101.

First Peoples' Cultural Council. (2018). Report on the status of B.C. First Nations languages. Retrieved February 15th from http://www.fpcc.ca/files/PDF/FPCC-LanguageReport-180716-WEB.pdf

Greenwood, M. & Leeuw, S. D. (2007). Teachings from the land: Indigenous people, our health. *Canadian Journal of Native Education*, *30*(1), 48–53.

Guilar, J. & Swallow, T. (2008). ÁLENENEC: Learning from place, spirit, and traditional language. *The Canadian Journal of Native Studies*, *28*(2), 273–293.

Iseke, J. (2013). Spirituality as decolonizing: Elders Albert Desjarlais, George McDermott, and Tom McCallum share understandings of life in healing practices. *Decolonization: Indigeneity, Education & Society*, *2*(1), 35–54.

Iseke-Barnes, J. M. (2008). Pedagogies for decolonizing. *Canadian Journal of Native Education*, *31*(1), 123–148.

Lavallee, L. F. & Poole, J. M. (2010). Beyond recovery: Colonization, health and healing for indigenous people in Canada. *International Journal of Mental Health and Addiction*, *8*(2), 271–281.

Louie, D. W., Poitras-Pratt, Y., Hanson, A. J., & Ottmann, J. (2017). Applying indigenizing principles of decolonizing methodologies in university classrooms. *Canadian Journal of Higher Education/Revue canadienne d'enseignement supérieur*, *47*(3), 16–33.

Meyer, M. A. (2008). Indigenous and authentic: Hawaiian epistemology and the triangulation of meaning. In N. K. Denzin, Y. S. Lincoln, & L. T. Smith

(Eds.), *Handbook of critical and indigenous methodologies* (pp. 217–232). Newberry Park, CA: Sage.

Morgensen, S. L. (2011). The biopolitics of settler colonialism: Right here, right now. *Settler Colonial Studies*, *1*(1), 52–76.

National Indian Brotherhood. (1972). Indian control of Indian education: A policy paper presented to the Minister of Indian Affairs and Northern Development. Retrieved from https://oneca.com/IndianControlofIndianEducation.pdf

Regan, P. (2010). *Unsettling the settler within: Indian residential schools, truth telling, and reconciliation in Canada*. Vancouver, Canada: UBC Press.

Ritchie, S. D., Wabano, M. J., Corbiere, R. G., Restoule, B. M., Russell, K. C., & Young, N. L. (2015). Connecting to the Good Life through outdoor adventure leadership experiences designed for indigenous youth. *Journal of Adventure Education and Outdoor Learning*, *15*(4), 350–370.

Simpson, L. R. (2004). Anticolonial strategies for the recovery and maintenance of indigenous knowledge. *American Indian Quarterly*, *28*(3/4), 373–384.

Simpson, L. B. (2014). Land as pedagogy: Nishnaabeg intelligence and rebellious transformation. *Decolonization: Indigeneity, Education & Society*, *3*(3), 1–25.

Statistics Canada. (2006). Aboriginal peoples in Canada in 2006: Inuit, Métis and First Nations, 2006 census. Retrieved from https://www12.statcan.gc.ca/census-recensement/2006/as-sa/97-558/pdf/97-558-XIE2006001.pdf

Truth and Reconciliation Commission of Canada. (2015). *Truth and reconciliation commission of Canada: Calls to action*. Winnipeg, Canada: Truth and Reconciliation Commission of Canada.

Tuck, E. & McKenzie, M. (2015). *Place in research, theory, methodology and methods*. New York, NY: Routledge.

Tuck, E. & Yang, K. W. (2012). Decolonization is not a metaphor. *Decolonization: Indigeneity, Education & Society*, *1*(1), 1–40.

Turner, N. J. & Hebda, R. (2012). *Saanich ethnobotany: Culturally important plants of the WSÁNEC people*. Victoria, Canada: Royal British Columbia Museum.

Turner, N. J., Lepofsky, D., & Deur, D. (2013). Plant management systems of British Columbia's first peoples. *BC Studies: The British Columbian Quarterly*, *179*, 107–133.

United Nations. (2007). *The United Nations declaration on the rights of indigenous peoples*. New York, NY: United Nations.

Williams, L., Bunda, T., Claxton, N., & MacKinnon, I. (2018). A global decolonial praxis of sustainability—Undoing epistemic violences between indigenous peoples and those no longer indigenous to place. *The Australian Journal of Indigenous Education*, *47*(1), 41–53.

Part II

Practices

Chapter 6

Wilderness Therapy

Carina Ribe Fernee and Leiv Einar Gabrielsen

Wilderness therapy is an experiential approach to mental health treatment combining the restorative qualities of nature with individual and group-based therapeutic processes (Davis-Berman & Berman, 2008; Russell, 2001). Ecological, physical, and psychosocial health dimensions together make up a holistic intervention. Venturing into the wild ideally involves a disconnection from technology and the slowing down from a hectic, urban existence. The group treatment may provide the time and space to begin a recovery process where relationships are built with the self, others, and the natural world. Wilderness therapy practice is diverse, ranging from structured, leader-directed approaches, to dynamic processes that are co-created between the participants, facilitators, and the natural environment.

Historical and Cultural Perspectives

In the United States, youth camping programs and experiential education are commonly referred to as the predecessors of wilderness therapy (Davis-Berman & Berman, 2008). In countries like Canada and Australia, influential traditions are Indigenous perspectives (see Chapter 5) and a strong connection to land (Harper, Gabrielsen, & Carpenter, 2018); while in the Scandinavian countries, a deep affiliation with nature and the simple life outdoors are essential in the *friluftsliv* tradition (Fernee, Gabrielsen, Andersen, & Mesel, 2015). The development of wilderness therapy across a range of socio-cultural contexts and traditions is expressed in the great diversity represented in the field today (Norton, Carpenter, & Pryor, 2015).

Target Populations and Key Developments

Wilderness therapy serves primarily youth and young adult populations, most commonly providing care for emotional, behavioral, psychological, and/or substance use problems (Hoag, Massey, & Roberts, 2014). Many programs integrate family work and some include local communities in the treatment process to anchor positive changes and fostering protective factors in the home environments (Norton, 2011).

Wilderness therapy can be provided as preventative or enrichment interventions in school- or community-based settings, and as a targeted primary treatment. It may serve as an adjunct to other services or be offered as a stand-alone intervention. Although wilderness therapy takes many forms, it continues to grow in visibility as a promising treatment option (Becker & Russell, 2016), although has not gained formal recognition in the continuum of youth mental health services (Berman & Davis-Berman, 2013).

Networking and collaboration are widespread across local, regional, and international forums (Norton et al., 2015). Considerations of theoretical conceptualization, therapeutic factors, along with professional and ethical standards are receiving increased attention (Becker & Russell, 2016). Substantial differences are found among the ways in which wilderness therapy programs are developed, implemented, and evaluated (Becker & Russell, 2016). Moving forward as a profession, this diversity must be negotiated and reconciled if our goal is to arrive at an integrative wilderness therapy practice.

We use this chapter to elaborate on what we see as future challenges which we will discuss throughout. However, we reiterate that as Norwegian authors we represent a particular perspective on the practice of wilderness therapy.

Discussion of Practice

Core Elements

Three main therapeutic factors have been proposed to make up core elements of the wilderness therapy treatment process, which is the combination of time spent in wilderness, the physical self, and the psychosocial self (Fernee, Gabrielsen, Andersen, & Mesel, 2017; Russell & Farnum, 2004). These core elements interact and are hardly separable. They do, however, illustrate the multidimensionality of nature-based group treatments.

The *natural environment* is important as both a treatment context and co-facilitator in wilderness therapy (Harper et al., 2018). Nature provides a novel and neutral therapeutic setting that can open up for new experiences, perspectives, and alternative ways of being or becoming (Hill, 2007; Williams, 2000). Harper, Rose, and Segal (2019) proposed the natural environment has calming qualities that can reduce stress and provide restoration. The therapists can step back from traditional positions of authority and let nature provide a therapeutic milieu where change is not forced, but rather evolves over time (Russell, 2001).

The second factor, *the physical self*, refers to the physical mobilization and the various tasks and challenges inherent to wilderness therapy.

Outdoor activities offer opportunities for experiential learning, personal growth, and mastery (Russell & Farnum, 2004), for instance, through managing the changing conditions and physical demands whilst hiking (Caulkins, White, & Russell, 2006). The importance of frequently assessing each participant's physical and emotional safety and well-being has been reiterated throughout the wilderness therapy literature (Davis-Berman & Berman, 2002; Gabrielsen, Harper, & Fernee, 2019).

The third core element, *the psychosocial self*, refers to the opportunities for developing self-insight, along with fostering a sense of belonging and connection over time, to peers, the therapists, and to nature. In wilderness therapy, facilitators are to approach the therapeutic relationship in a nurturing, caring, and empathetic way (Russell, 2001). Wilderness living demands cooperation and communication, where participants have the chance to help others and to practice altruism (Norton, 2011). Although exchanges of support can be intricate and not necessarily straightforward to navigate at all times (Fernee, Mesel, Andersen, & Gabrielsen, 2019).

Description of Techniques

Beyond the simple life outdoors and the intentional use of structured individual- and group-based therapy, other techniques include experiential exercises where nature is often an integrated part. Examples include, for instance, the use of natural elements as therapeutic metaphors. The natural consequences experienced by participants can symbolize the random occurrence of real-life events, which challenges youth to develop and make use of a variety of skill sets according to the changing conditions (Russell, 2006). Facilitated quiet time can encourage states of introspection and contemplation, where journal assignments can assist the reflection process (Norton, 2011). Outdoor activities provide opportunities for concrete accomplishments and mastery, whether it involves catching a fish, building a camp fire, or managing without access to social media, through which participants may come to realize previously 'hidden' abilities, resources, and alternative coping mechanisms.

Philosophical Underpinnings of Wilderness Therapy

Wilderness therapy takes place in nature, and arguably the more 'wild' this nature is—meaning unaltered by, and distant from humans—the better. The predominant explanation for nature's role in wilderness therapy is biological (Selhub & Logan, 2012). Humans have evolved in outdoor environments and survived as a species through our ability to adapt to it. Nature is *who we are* and this understanding of humans as non-dichotomous to nature lies at the core of philosophical approaches, such as deep ecology (Drengson & Devall, 2008) and ecosophy (Naess & Rothenberg, 1989), which in turn inform ecopsychology perspectives (Roszak, Gomes, & Kanner, 1995). Similar ecopsychological perspectives were explored in Chapter 3. All these approaches argue that the health and well-being of the natural world is intrinsically interwoven with the health and well-being of humans. This understanding permeates wilderness therapy as well. As most people in the industrialized world live in urban environments, we endure lifestyles that may be socially and culturally expected of us, but not that we are biologically adapted to. This, Louv (2008) proposed, may lead to conditions of increased alienation and meaninglessness, heightening the risk of physical and emotional struggles. The antidote for this maladaptation or *disease* being obvious; more time spent in contact with the natural world (Gabrielsen & Harper, 2018).

Theory, Research, and Efficacy

Outcome Studies

Although research within the field of wilderness therapy has improved over the last two decades and outcome studies have begun to provide evidence of efficacy, there remain limitations in terms of scope, depth, and methodological sophistication (Hoag et al., 2014). Overall, empirical publications on wilderness therapy support the notion of effectiveness in treatment of a broad range of social, emotional, and substance use issues (Harper, 2017). Reductions in clinical symptomatology, along with improvements in life effectiveness, self-esteem, locus of control, and interpersonal skills have been reported (Bettmann, Gillis, Speelman, Parry, & Case, 2016; Dobud & Harper, 2018; Hoag, Massey, Roberts, & Logan, 2013; Pryor, 2018), and positive outcomes are suggested to be sustained over time (Bowen & Neill, 2013; Combs, Hoag, Javorski, & Roberts, 2016).

Despite promising results, outcome studies typically include relatively small sample sizes, which limit the possibilities for statistical explorations, such as investigating comparison or subgroups. Furthermore, wilderness therapy programs vary with regard to populations served, duration, content, and outcome goals (Becker & Russell, 2016). Therefore, we should be cautious when generalizing findings from single studies onto the field at large.

A clearer understanding of how positive changes come about has been requested (Hoag et al., 2014), whereby researchers are encouraged to dig deeper to investigate why, how, and for whom wilderness therapy treatment appears to be helpful (Bettmann, Russell, & Parry, 2013).

Qualitative Understandings

In order to arrive at a more in-depth understanding and conceptualization of the wilderness therapy process, qualitative work often makes use of participant observation and interviews to investigate treatment experiences and perceived outcomes. Being in nature has been found to invoke reflexivity, improve moods, and clearing the mind, while reducing rumination (Conlon, Wilson, Gaffney, & Stoker, 2018; McIver, Senior, & Francis, 2018). Through time spent in nature, participants are proposed to gain "a more holistic perspective of who they are and what they can achieve, beyond preconceived notions and self-imposed labels" (McIver et al., 2018, p. 398). Wilderness therapy may open more avenues for mental health work, where participants feel freer, less confined, less 'crazy,' and 'in treatment' when compared to more conventional treatment settings (Conlon et al., 2018; Fernee et al., 2019).

In an Irish study, McIver and colleagues (2018) described what seemed to be an unfolding mind-body connection emerging out of the physicality of the treatment process. The experiential nature of wilderness therapy appears to provide a pathway from surface to deep knowledge (McIver et al., 2018), where new insights may enable self-awareness and self-regulation to emerge over time (Fernee, 2019).

In an Australian study, Conlon and colleagues (2018) reiterated the importance of the adolescent participants experiencing choice and control over their own situation in the wilderness. Feeling heard, valued, and cared for by the wilderness leaders conditioned participant engagement. This element of perceived influence was suggested to predispose the adolescents to not rebel from the program, but instead to remain open, interested, and grateful for the opportunity to participate in a nature-based group treatment and what they deemed to be a fun and novel experience.

Wilderness therapy involves opportunities for connecting with one's self, with others and with nature. Relational experiences may be restructured or strengthened in nature as the participants and facilitators spend time together in a wilderness context, endure the same conditions, share meals, and get to know each other. Such relational dynamics appear to be at the core of the healing process (Norton, 2011).

A number of these aspects come into play in the story of a young boy, here called Espen, who participated in a Norwegian wilderness therapy program called *friluftsterapi*, or "therapy in the open air" (Fernee et al., 2015). This outdoor group treatment seemed to provide the time and space Espen needed in order to reconnect with his emotions and begin a process of grief, which appeared to be supported by the alliances that arose in the outdoors.

Case Vignette: The Time and Space to Heal Naturally

Espen was a tall and lean 17-year-old boy. His long blond hair was kept in place beneath a colorful beanie. His handshake was firm and he came across as a polite, considerate, and overall very likeable person. He was however struggling immensely, ever since his father passed away two years earlier. Overnight, 15-year-old Epsen took on increased responsibilities in the household that now consisted of only himself and his grieving mother. Over time, he developed symptoms of depression, accompanied by low self-esteem and self-worth. His motivation and school performance declined rapidly. Bullying increased and added to the load he was already carrying on his young shoulders, Espen remained in bed most days. A tragedy of two youngsters from Espen's school committing suicide only a few days apart in the nearby forest area, quickly accelerated the concern as Espen had expressed suicidal ideation to a friend of the family. Espen agreed to be referred to mental health services at the local hospital, upon which he was informed of available treatment options; one of them being wilderness therapy.

At the time, five aspects of an outdoor treatment seemed to be particularly well aligned with Espen's situation and preferences. First, he proclaimed that there was "no chance in hell" that he would sit in an office and talk about his struggles. Second, while living in an urban suburb the latter years, Espen grew up in the countryside and nature was his playground. The fondest memories of his deceased father were the many outdoor activities they had shared. Third, Espen could use some time away from his home environment. He felt like a burden on his mother and hated school. Fourth, his low self-worth made him question his social abilities and he had become skeptical toward peers and adults alike. Although he dreaded it, Espen realized the need to relate to people his age and felt like the outdoors were the safest milieu to do it in. Finally, the slow pace of our wilderness therapy approach (friluftsterapi) allowed for relational and emotional processes to evolve naturally, whilst initial insecurity could subside at its own pace.

In many ways Espen was a typical wilderness therapy participant. Despite feeling mentally and physically fatigued at the onset of the intervention, the simple life outdoors was perceived to be an engaging environment. Espen's resourcefulness manifested quickly. However, when group therapy sessions were initiated, the long blond hair would partially cover his face and his remarks remained equally unrevealing. After spending three days together in an outdoor camp to learn skills, a basic level of trust was established within the group. Espen told us in retrospect, he had realized that the other youth and therapists were prepared to accompany him into, metaphorically speaking, more demanding terrain.

Wilderness therapy can be an unpredictable and dynamic approach to treatment, where unplanned moments can turn out to be the most significant moments of change. On the second overnight trip, coincidences led Espen and one of the male therapists to hike separately from the rest of the group for a couple of hours. The route was demanding and the therapist had filled his backpack to the rim with equipment needed for transitioning between campsites. By now, Espen had strengthened his physical stamina, striding seemingly effortlessly like a moose on his long legs through the wet and soggy forest terrain. The therapist, on the other hand, was not comfortable with Espen's pace and during a break seized the opportunity inherent in the situation and admitted, "Espen, I'm not having my best of days, would you mind helping me by taking some of the load from my backpack?" Espen immediately responded by taking a tent and some of the food from the therapist's to his own backpack.

This simple act initiated an alliance that was further developed as the two of them cooperated on navigating by map and compass en route to the campsite by the lake mid-forest. The hike became more than a transit from one campsite to the next.

The two shared stories of past times spent in the outdoors, and equally important moments in silence. Espen had a keen eye for details and at one point spotted a nest of grouse eggs. Gently approaching the nest he quietly uttered, "I found a nest of eggs, much like this one, with my father not so long ago." Espen did not cry, but looked the therapist firmly in the eyes and the significance of this moment shared between the two somewhere mid-forest was inevitable. The discovery seemed to ignite a more proactive stance from Espen, as if this was the sign he had been waiting for in order to devote himself wholeheartedly to the process.

As the two of them arrived at the campsite in the late afternoon, the shimmering surface of the forest lake faded as the sun descended behind the pine trees in the horizon. The tents were pitched, firewood gathered and dinner was prepared. As the cool Nordic night shortly engulfed the group, they gathered closely around the campfire. Jokes and laughter were as frequent as existential reflections and soul-searching questions. Espen kept the fire going until late that night. Too late some would argue. While others gradually resigned to their sleeping bags, Espen and Anne, two youngsters who both had experienced their unfair share of hardship in life, remained under the star sign of Cassiopeia. The flickering lights from the campfire played on the canvas of the tents that surrounded them, accompanied by the calm voices in the night as the two shared their stories unfiltered and uninterrupted.

Reflecting back on his experiences of treatment, Espen recalled this particular day and night as forever memorable. He emphasized how he gradually came to see the therapists and the peers as persons he could confide in, who could support him onto a path toward a life that felt worth living. The story of Espen reminds us of what can be the essence of wilderness therapy: the multitude of connections that can arise, the resources that can emerge, and the stories that can be shared, adjusted, and co-created when provided the time and space to grow naturally.

Discussion

Wilderness therapy is practiced across the globe on Canadian rivers, Israeli deserts, Finnish forests, Icelandic mountains, and in the Australian bush. The variations that are deemed to be found across contexts are in principle of great value, however may also require us to dialogue on those times where our cultures and traditions may cause us to view matters differently. Such conversations can be demanding and at times upsetting; yet willingness to engage in collaborative professional and ethical reflections are important and necessary if we want to continue down a common path moving forward.

In our humble opinion there are, and in addition to numerous expected smaller obstacles, two major hindrances lie ahead for the field of wilderness therapy: the climate crisis and relational dignity. One of these challenges is unfortunately not something we as a field will be able to resolve, but that we should still respond proactively to.

Climate Crisis

As an outdoor therapy, we must come to understand that all practitioners affiliated with wilderness therapy should acknowledge our environmental responsibility. This stance is not only moral in itself, but also serves as logical consequence of the human-nature reciprocal relationship. We live in an epoch labeled the Anthropocene in which humans are dramatically transforming the planet. We should take it upon ourselves to be nature's guardians and spokespersons, where immediate implications should be to conduct our work and lead our lives with as little environmental impact as possible. In addition, strive to raise environmental awareness wherever we go. This discussion is continued in Part 3 of this book.

Relational Dignity

The second potential challenge on our path moving forward is the standing of the wilderness therapy field if we do not uphold a standard of *relational dignity* in all facets of our practice. Moving forward, in-depth conversations could entail how we can understand, and in all situations attempt to uphold, the concept of relational dignity or equivalent terms. What does it entail across contexts and how does it hold up against the end justifies the means argument? Are we as a field ready to consider whether everything that is practiced en route to, or in, wilderness therapy today foster feelings of autonomy, empowerment, and self-worth in our participants? This topic is of utmost importance, not only for afflicted vulnerable youth but also for the standing of our field in the eyes of the public.

A topic that ties closely to relational dignity is the prevalence of coercion in some wilderness therapy programs (Harper, 2017; Tucker et al., 2018). Compulsory treatment may at times be warranted, but we have to ask ourselves, particularly due to the context of wilderness therapy and working where no one can see us, how we can possibly ensure the highest ethical standard in our practice. Arguably, two programs, one where the participants cannot leave, the other where the client can terminate the treatment at any time he or she chooses, operate in very different ways, particularly with regard to client-therapist relations. In plain, they are fundamentally different approaches to treatment.

If you are new to this field, working in the wilderness with the aim to support participants' recovery, development, and growth can be a personally deeply rewarding experience. Being outdoors removes much of the control, predictability, and structures found in indoor environments, whereby practitioners who are happy to improvise as the intervention unfolds will not only be the most comfortable, but arguably also those providing the best care.

As with other treatment approaches, wilderness therapy should be purposeful, collaborative, and based on a thorough participant assessment and individualized treatment plan. Furthermore, each participant's level of comfort must be monitored, along with a consideration of which outdoor activities may serve their best interests, where the overall principle is to do no harm. Facilitators must therefore ensure that they are mindful of practicing within their boundaries of competence. According to Reese (2016) "The more specific the activity, the more remote the location, and greater the physical or psychological risk, the more specific training and expertise the counselor must maintain to ensure client safety in outdoor contexts" (p. 350). When we feel safe, cared for, and at ease in nature, we will unconditionally share the inherent joy, peacefulness, and gratitude as we connect at a deeper level. Provided the time and space to do so, we may restore our relationships with ourselves, with others, and with nature, whereby experiencing healing in a relational context as we venture together into the wild.

References

Becker, S. P. & Russell, K. C. (2016). Wilderness therapy. In R. J. R. Levesque (Ed.), *Encyclopedia of adolescence* (2nd ed., pp. 1–10). Cham, Switzerland: Springer International.

Berman, D. S. & Davis-Berman, J. (2013). The role of therapeutic adventure in meeting the mental health needs of children and adolescents: Finding a niche in the health care systems of the United States and the United Kingdom. *Journal of Experiential Education, 36*, 51–64.

Bettmann, J. E., Gillis, H. L., Speelman, E. A., Parry, K. J., & Case, J. M. (2016). A Meta-analysis of wilderness therapy outcomes for private pay clients. *Journal of Child and Family Studies, 25*, 2659–2673.

Bettmann, J. E., Russell, K. C., & Parry, K. J. (2013). How substance abuse recovery skills, readiness to change and symptom reduction impact change processes in wilderness therapy participants. *Journal of Child and Family Studies, 12*, 1039–1050.

Bowen, D. J. & Neill, J. T. (2013). A meta-analysis of adventure therapy outcomes and moderators. *The Open Psychology Journal, 6*, 28–53.

Caulkins, M. C., White, D. D., & Russell, K. C. (2006). The role of physical exercise in wilderness therapy for troubled adolescent women. *Journal of Experiential Education, 29*, 18–37.

Combs, K. M., Hoag, M. J., Javorski, S., & Roberts, S. D. (2016). Adolescent self-assessment of an outdoor behavioral health program: Longitudinal outcomes and trajectories of change. *Journal of Child and Family Studies, 25*, 3322–3330.

Conlon, C. M., Wilson, C. E., Gaffney, P., & Stoker, M. (2018). Wilderness therapy intervention with adolescents: Exploring the process of change. *Journal of Adventure Education and Outdoor Learning, 18*, 353–366.

Davis-Berman, J. & Berman, D. (2002). Risk and anxiety in adventure programming. *Journal of Experiential Education, 25*, 305–310.

Davis-Berman, J. & Berman, D. S. (1994). *Wilderness therapy: Foundations, theory & research*. Dubuque, IA: Kendall/Hunt Publishing.

Davis-Berman, J. & Berman, D. S. (2008). *The promise of wilderness therapy*. Boulder, CO: Association for Experiential Education.

Dobud, W. & Harper, N. J. (2018). Of dodo birds and common factors: A scoping review of direct comparison trials in adventure therapy. *Complementary Therapies in Clinical Practice, 31*, 16–24.

Drengson, A. & Devall, B. (2008). *The ecology of wisdom. Writings by Arne Naess*. Berkeley, CA: Publishers Group West.

Fernee, C. R. (2019). Into nature. A realist exploration of wilderness therapy in adolescent mental health care in Norway. Doctoral Dissertation. Kristiansand, Norway: University of Agder.

Fernee, C. R., Gabrielsen, L. E., Andersen, A. J. W., & Mesel, T. (2015). Therapy in the open air: Introducing wilderness therapy to the adolescent mental health services in Scandinavia. *Scandinavian Psychologist, 2*, e14.

Fernee, C. R., Gabrielsen, L. E., Andersen, A. J. W., & Mesel, T. (2017). Unpacking the black box of wilderness therapy: A realist synthesis. *Qualitative Health Research, 21*, 114–129.

Fernee, C. R., Mesel, T., Andersen, A. J. W., & Gabrielsen, L. E. (2019). Therapy the natural way: A realist exploration of the wilderness therapy treatment process in adolescent mental health care in Norway. *Qualitative Health Research, 29*, 1358–1377.

Gabrielsen, L. E. & Harper, N. J. (2018). The role of wilderness therapy in the face of global trends of urbanization and technification. *International Journal of Adolescence and Youth, 23*, 409–421.

Gabrielsen, L. E., Harper, N. J., & Fernee, C. R. (2019). What are constructive anxiety levels in wilderness therapy? An exploratory pilot study. *Complementary Therapies in Clinical Practice, 37*, 51–57.

Harper, N. J. (2017). Wilderness therapy, therapeutic camping and adventure education in child and youth care literature: A scoping review. *Children and Youth Services Review, 83*, 68–79.

Harper, N. J., Gabrielsen, L. E., & Carpenter, C. (2018). Cross-cultural exploration of 'wild' in wilderness therapy: Canadian, Australian and Norwegian perspectives. *Journal of Adventure Education and Outdoor Learning, 18*, 148–164.

Harper, N. J., Rose, K., & Segal, D. (2019). *Nature-based therapy. A practitioner's guide to working outdoors with children, youth, and families.* Gabriola Island, Canada: New Society Publishers.

Hill, N. R. (2007). Wilderness therapy as a treatment modality for at-risk youth: A primer for mental health counselors. *Journal of Mental Health Counseling, 29*, 338–349.

Hoag, M. J., Massey, K., & Roberts, S. D. (2014). Dissecting the wilderness therapy client: Examining clinical trends, findings, and patterns. *Journal of Experiential Education, 37*, 382–396.

Hoag, M. J., Massey, K., Roberts, S. D., & Logan, P. (2013). Efficacy of wilderness therapy for young adults: A first look. *Residential Treatment for Children and Youth, 30*, 294–305.

Louv, R. (2008). *Last child in the woods: Saving our children from nature-deficit disorder.* Chapel Hill, NC: Algonquin Books.

McIver, S., Senior, E., & Francis, Z. (2018). Healing fears, conquering challenges: Narrative outcomes from a wilderness therapy program. *Journal of Creativity in Mental Health, 13*, 392–404.

Naess, A. & Rothenberg, D. (1989). *Ecology, community and lifestyle.* Cambridge, MA: Cambridge University Press.

Norton, C. L. (2011). Wilderness therapy: Creating a context of hope. In Norton, C. L. (Ed.), *Innovative interventions in child and adolescent mental health.* (pp. 48–86) New York, NY: Routledge.

Norton, C. L., Carpenter, C., & Pryor, A. (Eds). (2015). *Adventure therapy around the globe: International perspectives and diverse approaches.* Champaign, IL: Common Ground Publishing LLC.

Pryor, A. (2018). *Outdoor adventure interventions–Young people and adversity: A literature review.* Richmond, Australia: Berry Street Victoria Inc.

Reese, R. F. (2016). EcoWellness & guiding principles for the ethical integration of nature into counseling. *International Journal of Adventure Counselling, 38*, 345–357.

Roszak, T., Gomes, M. A., & Kanner, A. D. (1995). *Ecopsychology.* San Fransisco, CA: Sierra Club Books.

Russell, K. C. (2001). What is wilderness therapy? *Journal of Experiential Education, 24*, 70–79.

Russell, K. C. (2006). Brat camp, boot camp, or …? Exploring wilderness therapy program theory. *Journal of Adventure Education and Outdoor Learning, 6*, 51–68.

Russell, K. C. & Farnum, J. (2004). A concurrent model of the wilderness therapy process. *Journal of Adventure Education and Outdoor Learning, 4*, 39–55.

Selhub, E. M. & Logan, A. C. (2012). *Your brain on nature. The science of nature's influence on your health, happiness, and vitality.* Mississauga, Canada: Wiley Canada.

Tucker, A. R., Combs, K. M., Bettmann, J. E., Chang, T-H., Graham, S., Hoag, M., & Tatum, C. (2018). Longitudinal outcomes for youth transported to wilderness therapy programs. *Research on Social Work Practice, 28*, 438–451.

Williams, B. (2000). The treatment of adolescent populations: An institutional vs. a wilderness setting. *Journal of Child and Adolescent Group Therapy, 10*, 47–56.

Chapter 7

Adventure Therapy

Cathryn Carpenter and Anita Pryor

Introduction and Background

The depiction of adventure resonates throughout literature, oral histories, and folklore, from Homer's Odyssey to tales of modern expeditions, and adventure has been attributed to human growth and development (Hopkins & Putnam, 2013). Centering adventure within a therapeutic construct enables practitioners and participants to access the values and health benefits of nature contact through encounters with risk, challenge, and new horizons. Mortlock (1987) wrote:

> To adventure in the natural environment is consciously to take up a challenge that will demand the best of our capabilities - physically, mentally and emotionally. It is a state of mind that will initially accept unpleasant feelings of fear, uncertainty and discomfort, and the need for luck, because we instinctively know that, if we are successful, these will be counterbalanced by opposite feelings of exhilaration and joy.
>
> (p. 19)

Of Latin origins, the word 'adventure' includes notions of ad, venio, and advento, in which *ad* means "a direction towards, an extension, a motion," *venio* means a metaphorical movement "to arise, to grow," and *advent* means "to approach, to proceed onwards, to advance" (Simpson, 1991; White & Oxen, 1893). Pryor (2009) suggested "these definitions hint at the dynamic therapeutic potential within the ancient roots of the word adventure" (p. 28).

The contemporary field of adventure therapy has been described as many tribal groups, reflecting different schools of thought and practice (Harper, Peeters, & Carpenter, 2014; Ringer, 2003). In recent years, the global field of International Adventure Therapy has come to encompass the various tribes:

> As indicated by the name, the two core elements of adventure therapy are: (1) engagement in adventurous (physical) activities;

and (2) therapeutic intent. Beyond this, we must consider the social, cultural, environmental, political and fiscal contexts that influence the development of local adventure therapy practices.

(IAT, 2019a, para. 3)

This chapter outlines key mechanisms and ethical considerations at work within adventure therapy and provides a snapshot of theories and research that highlight therapeutic benefits. A case study illustrates practice, and a final discussion offers a sample of current and future trends. The intentional use of adventure within outdoor therapies is both challenging and exciting. Supporting human capacities to endure and succeed is at the heart of this approach.

Discussion of Practice

Adventure therapy mobilizes four key mechanisms to elicit therapeutic change (Pryor, Pryor, & Carpenter, 2018), which can provide an immersive therapeutic environment, from which participants can gain multiple benefits:

- Physical experiences of challenge and adventure
- Therapeutic support and intentional conversations
- Social experiences of connecting with others
- Ecological experiences in natural environments

Physical Experiential Adventures

Recent definitions of adventure include notions of risk, challenge, and danger (e.g., Ayto, 1990); or "an unusual, exciting and possibly dangerous activity" (Cambridge English Dictionary, 2019). Globally, adventure therapy services use physical activities as a way of engaging participants' physical, mental, and emotional selves in the therapeutic experience (Gass, Gillis, & Russell, 2012). In some places, adventure activities are the 'therapy'; in other settings, activities are used to support therapeutic processes and outcomes. In Australia, adventure therapy provides "challenges of the mind, body and spirit, for people of all cultures, genders, ages, stages and identities" (AABAT, 2019, n.p.).

The design and use of physical activities can be relatively simple yet a range of initiatives have occurred in practice, like walking through bushland to explore sense of self in a place, through to a highly structured and prescribed activity, like doing a ropes course for mental health treatment. Adventure experiences can range from one-off 'taster' experiences to a programmed sequence of events that gain intensity over time, to extended multi-day journeys.

Activities can be relaxed, with perceptions of danger relatively low, or highly physically challenging, where dangers are real. Group-based adventure activities must take into account the needs of all individuals within the group. What is a safe 'adventure' for one participant may be experienced as 'misadventure' for another. No matter the level of challenge, it is important that activities feel attainable to a participant, and provide authentic and clear consequences for decisions and actions or inactions taken (Deane & Harré, 2014; Harper et al., 2014).

Therapeutic Support and Intentional Conversations

In the United States, 'adventure therapists' are expected to hold a graduate level degree in a mental health field (AEE, 2019). In Australia, adventure therapy practice includes general therapeutic outcomes as well as the specific intent of therapy (AABAT, 2019), so practitioners tend to work in cross-disciplinary teams and may hold diverse qualifications in social work, psychology, youth work, and teaching among others.

Regardless of training, adventure therapists and practitioners should be aware of the possibility that participants have experienced previous trauma, and understand how to build safe and therapeutic relationships (Kezelman & Stavropoulos, 2019). Being trauma-informed can help practitioners avoid triggering traumatic memories or enactments in participants (Norton, Wisner, Krugh, & Penn, 2014).

The strong therapeutic alliance developed between practitioners and participants is a defining element of all therapy, including adventure therapy (Harper, 2009). While some practitioners provide planned counselling sessions in a structured way during an adventure, others provide useful conversations more seamlessly. In either case, the client to practitioner relationship is usually democratized through the quality of shared challenges and bonding experiences (Pryor, Conway, & Pryor, 2019).

Social Connections

Group-based adventure therapy experiences are more common than one-to-one experiences (Gass et al., 2012). In some adventure therapy services, the group work is the therapy. In others settings, social relationships are simply part of the therapeutic milieu. Within Australia, adventure therapy has an overarching aim of increasing health and well-being for individuals, families, groups, and communities (AABAT, 2019), highlighting the importance of social relationships and a systemic approach.

The design and use of social relationships is often intentional and structured, for example, involving rigorous selection processes, pre-planned group sessions, a sequence of group tasks, and allocation of social roles and responsibilities. Across different practices, the development of social agreements is used to support social safety, and the establishment of strong attachments is a common goal, either within the program or with other significant people in participants' lives.

Ecological Experiences

Most adventure therapy interventions take place in outdoor environments. Nature is an ideal setting for adventure due to its novelty and appeal. In Australia, nature is often called 'bush,' a term that encompasses the whole range of natural environments, from small green spaces in urban settings to vast remote expanses of bushland or coast (Pryor, Carpenter, & Townsend, 2005).

Some practitioners view the immersion in nature as the 'therapy' while others from different traditions view nature as a co-therapist (Harper, Rose, & Segal, 2019). The outdoor setting may also be used simply as a venue or 'clinic' for conventional therapeutic practices, such as 'walk and talk' therapy (Jordan & Marshall, 2010). For some Indigenous and non-Indigenous people, adventure therapy involves returning home to areas of land or water inextricably linked with culture, sense of belonging, spiritual well-being, and health (Rae & Nichols, 2015; Ritchie et al., 2015).

While adventure therapy practitioners will likely understand the benefits of contact with nature, they are also expected to understand that novel environments can bring out different responses in participants, including possible triggering for those who have experienced previous trauma (Pryor et al., 2018).

Holistic Safetynet

Holistic safety in this dynamic therapeutic environment can be supported within by adhering to the ethical principles of a practitioner's stated profession (e.g., social work or psychology) or peak body (such as the British Association for Counselling and Psychotherapy's principles that may be used by practitioners in the UK), or by working to meet the ethical principles of adventure therapy bodies, such as those developed by the Therapeutic Adventure Professional Group (TAPG) in the United States (AEE, 2019) or the Australian Association for Bush Adventure Therapy (AABAT, 2019), as examples.

The Australian Association for Bush Adventure Therapy, Inc. (2019) provided a list of guiding principles that practitioners are encouraged to work toward:

- Positive regard for all people
- Respect for differences in culture, gender, age, and identity

- Strong family and community connections
- Transparency, informed consent, confidentiality
- Voluntary participation (within the confines of service type)
- Selection for 'readiness' to participate
- Attention to individual and group needs and hopes
- Supportive physical, psychological, and social environments
- Tailored adventure experiences
- Provision of options and choices (including supported exits)
- Respect for cultural custodianship of country
- Increasing self-awareness and reflexive practice
- No harm to self, others, or natural environments.

These ethical principles can be applied to all dimensions of an adventure therapy experience and ultimately result in programs that are closely attuned to providing the best possible therapeutic encounter for both the individual and the group. It is the needs of the target group, the intention of the service, and the skills and imagination of the staff team that lead to decisions within this approach.

Theory, Research, and Efficacy

Key Philosophies and Theories

The innate appeal of adventure is usually individual and subjective, which results in multiple philosophies and theories being used to explain therapeutic gains. According to Quin (1990), "To fly, wrapped in an impulse from the unknown towards the unknown, lies close to the heart of the experience of adventure" (p. 147). This subjectivity has led to the application of approaches that range from naturalistic and generative (Loynes, 2002) through to scientific and positivist (Crisp, 2004) and diverse practices around the world.

Fundamentally, "outdoor adventure activities are the primary practice of adventure therapy, while experiential learning methodologies guide its facilitation" (Harper et al., 2014, p. 225). When people have sought to articulate the concept of the adventure experience, early theories focused on matching the level of skill of the individual to the level of risk or challenge provided in the task or activity as a means of designing a peak adventure or optimal experience of 'flow' for participants (Csikszentmihalyi, 1975; Martin & Priest, 1986). These concepts are more recently described as a positive use of stress, or eustress, within this approach (Gass et al., 2012), though the intentional use of stress as received criticism from scholars, such as Mitten (1994). Chapter 14 explores these concepts in more depth.

The act of immersing oneself in a dynamic outdoor environment can be complex, especially when the intention is to achieve individual therapeutic outcomes in a group context. Prochaska, and DiClemente's (1982) 'Stages of change model' described the readiness of participants to engage in new activities and behaviors, and the successful pathway to maintain these changes. Bettmann, Russell, and Parry (2013), however, found reported readiness to change among adolescents in wilderness therapy programs did not affect positive outcomes. Still, this theory informs practitioners to meet the individual needs of participants rather than fitting individual needs into the service model.

The healing benefits of physical recreation and mastery support the empirical evidence of adventure therapy as a whole body and mind experience. For example, research by Perry (2006) and Jackson (2016) found that healing severe childhood adversities requires interventions that include physical activities; sensory integration promotion activities; psychological interventions (for new knowledge, skills, attitudes, and beliefs); social interventions (for new knowledge, skills, attitudes, and beliefs); systemic interventions (to support changes made); and environment-based interventions. Sensory integrative practice is discussed in greater detail in Chapter 11.

Through immersion in a natural place with a group of people, adventure therapy can lead to multiple therapeutic outcomes, such as improved well-being, self-esteem, and self-concept (Bowen & Neill, 2015). Providers are encouraged to search for and apply relevant research to their particular service to support safe and effective practice based on their given target group.

Research and Efficacy

To summarize, research that speaks to the diversity of adventure therapy aims and purpose, we return to four of the key mechanisms at work within adventure therapy and provide examples of research that contributes to our understanding of the benefits of adventure therapy across biological, psychological, social, and ecological domains of well-being.

- *Biological benefits* gained from physical and experiential activities include immediate physiological benefits, such as lowering of blood pressure, resetting circadian rhythms and longer term benefits in areas of physical fitness, outdoor skill development, physical competence and confidence, kinesthetic awareness, healthy eating, good nutrition, body care, and opportunities to reconnect physical and emotional experiences (Carpenter & Harper, 2016; Gladwell, Brown, Wood, Sandercock, & Barton, 2013; Tucker, Norton, DeMille, & Hobson, 2016).
- *Psychological benefits* include the fostering of mental health, resilience, self-efficacy, and mindfulness (Mutz & Müller, 2016), reducing

behavioral and emotional symptoms (Russell, 2003), raising self-esteem, courage, and levels of optimism about the future (Bowen & Neill, 2015), and inspiring movement from 'old me' to 'new me' (Knowles, 2013). Emotional benefits include lifting of spirits, improvements in self-concept (West & Crompton, 2001), and higher levels of other positive emotions such as happiness, pride, fun, hope, and satisfaction.

- *Social benefits* are one of the most commonly reported outcomes of adventure therapy, including the development of trust, increased understanding and acceptance of others, enhanced communication skills, greater social competence and confidence, and reduced isolation (Carpenter, Cameron, Cherednichenko, & Townsend, 2007; Holman & McAvoy, 2005), improved social and family well-being, improved attachment to parents, decreased anger toward parents (Bettmann & Tucker, 2011), and translation of newly developed social skills to other settings (Norton et al., 2014).
- *Ecological benefits* gained from adventure therapy include the range of mental, cultural, and spiritual benefits to be gained from physical activity in nature, along with potential benefits for nature itself, and natural environments including development of connection with life other than humans and sense of spiritual connectedness for both participants and practitioners.

Bowen and Neill's (2013) meta-analysis of adventure therapy outcomes and moderators found that adventure therapy programs tend to benefit participants socially, behaviorally, and psychologically. Furthermore, the meta-analysis provided strong evidence that these benefits of adventure therapy are comparable to the majority of efficacious treatments for patients across the age span reported in the literature. Given the significant and comparable findings for most categories of outcomes, the authors concluded that adventure therapy has broad application for adolescents and adults for a wide range of presenting issues.

Case Vignette: Regenerating Women and Children after Family Violence

On a three-day winter snow camp, five participating women were offered the opportunity to sleep in tents with their children in the snow. Two of the mothers took up the challenge. After dinner, these family groups were guided by staff to their tents under the light of a bright moon; the families adjusting to the frozen white world. One mother's experience of sleeping in the snow with her children turned out to be a significant turning point for her family. In the quiet stillness of the winter chill, and cocooned in the safety and privacy of a tent, she listened to her children talking for the first time about the abuses that had happened in their family. This sharing of stories between siblings was the first time any of them had put words to their experiences. It was the first sharing of shameful and fearful secrets that had lasted for years. The conversation established trust, and a new alliance between family members. For the mother, these tent-bound conversations felt like the start of new relationships in her family: "To build relations and trust with my kids, together again, was a blessing. We reunited… we were surrounded by lovely people who did not ask any questions, just were holding a space for us, it is so good."

Program Context and Client Group

A partnership between a women's refuge and an adventure therapy service provider led to the creation of a new adventure therapy service, which was the basis for a preliminary body of outcome research with this target group. A literature review identified 'common approaches' known to be important in supporting recovery from family violence, along with suitable tools to measure recovery progress (Pryor et al., 2018).

The recruitment of an all-female staff team with the skills and experience to implement the new service brought a mix of qualifications, including social work, general counselling, family therapy, community development, early childhood development, outdoor education, recreation, and leadership. Four of the five staff had previously worked in adventure therapy settings. All staff were provided with a five-day adventure therapy orientation, training in family violence, and trauma-informed care, individualized professional development, and regular professional supervision.

'Regenerate' Program Model

The intention of the Regenerate service model is to address the traumatic impacts of family violence by supporting the recovery of women and their children through adventure therapy. As with the wider international adventure therapy field, evidence-informed 'Mechanisms of Change' used within Regenerate include: (1) physical activities and use of adventure; (2) a therapeutic framework and counselling conversations; (3) a safe and supportive small group; and (4) contact with nature. The tailored combination of Regenerate's 'Mechanisms of Change' offers survivors a group-based 'environment of recovery.'

The Regenerate model offers a calendar of adventure therapy events including (a) two-hour adventure sessions; (b) whole-day adventures; (c) overnight adventure camps; (d) one-to-one counselling; and (e) celebration events. After an initial assessment and participation in a two-hour adventure session, all women can 'choose their own adventure' by selecting which events they would like to participate in, with or without children. The women are provided the opportunity to exit at any point, or maintain ongoing involvement for years.

Regenerate Practices

While informed by some of the evidence we have presented above and designed to be clinically safe, Regenerate is not 'clinical' in nature, and does not focus on the pathologies of participants. In practical terms, Regenerate offers a break from thinking about family violence experiences and the opportunity to reflect on life before and beyond family violence. The adventure therapy events take place in outdoor settings, from local parks in urban settings through to immersive experiences in remote bush, mountain, river, and ocean environments. The range of adventure activities include sitting quietly in nature, gentle group activities, such as walking, canoeing on flat or moving water, stand-up paddle boarding, abseiling, rock climbing, and snow camping, to name a few.

Program evaluation of processes and recovery outcomes for the participating women ($n = 196$) supported the importance of all four mechanisms of change while also illuminating a possible fifth: time for reflection and the emergence of personal insights (Rakar-Szabo, Steele, Smith, & Pryor, 2019). Thematic analysis indicated the women's favorite parts of the Regenerate adventure therapy service were the 'positive feelings' and 'sense of belonging' gained through 'physical adventures in nature with others' and 'opportunities to reflect.'

The most commonly cited recovery outcomes for children from the perspectives of their mothers were the development of healthy connections with other children and adults, greater family cohesion, reduction in conflicts with mothers and siblings, a better understanding of the causes of violence within family relationships, and helping to prevent family violence in the next generation. One woman said, "If I am self confident, my kids also will be better, and then we all will be safe, and can manage our life better" (Rakar-Szabo et al., 2019, p. 8). The detailed evaluation concluded, "Not only are survivors receiving therapeutic support by trained counsellors, they are experiencing adventurous physical activity and contact with nature led by trained [bush adventure therapy] practitioners, and the added benefits of authentic peer friendships" (Rakar-Szabo et al., 2019, p. 9).

Discussion

The field of adventure therapy is growing and gaining more credibility as a viable therapeutic approach around the globe (Norton et al., 2014).

With new approaches being developed in continental Europe, the Nordic region, Spain, New Zealand, and Hungary to name a few (IAT, 2019b), we should be aware of the global trends that will impact programs and practice. Significant current trends include the following:

- Increasing restrictions and limitations on accessing wild natural people-free places and the growing awareness of the benefits and increased use of local urban nature
- Growing sedentary culture and lifestyles with the associated reluctance to be active for the general population compared to global increases in bespoke adventure recreation and adventure tourism which is impacting on access to natural places with potential resource intensive/environmental harm
- Understanding that trauma underlies many behavioral and social problems—across the diversity of target populations and the need to tailor programs with flexible person-centered approaches and be more critical of how power is experienced within programs and by programs participants
- Outdoor therapy approaches can build health for people and all living organisms by influencing an increased understanding of climate change and the need for more protection of natural places

These trends have a range of implications for both practitioners in the field, and the development of research to deepen our understanding of how adventure therapy processes work and the range of outcomes these experiences can achieve. Implications include the need for multi-skilled practitioners and/or multi-disciplinary teams importance of self-aware reflexive practitioners. Questions also exist in how to train adventure therapy practitioners in a realistic and affordable time frame so they can enter the field with a breadth of skills and knowledge (Pryor, 2015). The diversity of programs and processes internationally limits opportunities for meta evaluations, meta-analysis, and systematic or narrative reviews. Adventure therapy approaches make research difficult to isolate the components, such as for random control experiments (Gabrielsen, Fernee, Aasen, & Eskedal, 2016). In this case, we feel evidence-informed practice more useful than evidence-based practice (Dobud, 2017). The use of adventure can de-stigmatize and de-medicalize therapy leading the dominant forms of medical research to be challenged by adventure therapy programs. Finally, programs should consciously connect with the communities and environments in their local region to strengthen the ongoing sustainability of the health and well-being of the entire community (e.g., centering of Indigenous peoples and knowledges in practice).

Conclusion

Nurturing a sense of curiosity keeps us alive. Seeking to make things better, to live a fulfilling life, and having the willingness to venture into the unknown is important for the sustainability of our future. Adventure encourages us to try new things, challenge ourselves, push our understandings of what we are individually and collectively capable of, and take responsibility for personal growth and development. Adventures in body, spirit, and mind can sustain the soul and lead to healthier individuals and communities if we are willing to include them within our lives. As Quin stated;

> without actively seeking, without attempting to and going beyond what one already knows one can accomplish there is no growth ... where there is no growth, where stagnation is the rule, a human being offers nothing, either to one's self or to society. (p. 147).

References

Association for Experiential Education [AEE]. (2019). *Adventure therapy best practices: Practitioner roles in adventure therapy*. Downloaded from the AEE/TAPG website October 2019. https://www.aee.org/tapg-best-p-practitioner-roles

Australian Association for Bush Adventure Therapy [AABAT]. (2019). *Bush Adventure Therapy 101: AABAT Training Workshop handbook*. Australian Association for Bush Adventure Therapy, Inc.

Ayto, J. (1990). *Bloomsbury dictionary of word origins*. New York, NY: Arcade Publishing.

Bettmann, J. E. & Tucker, A. R. (2011). Shifts in attachment relationships: A study of adolescents in wilderness treatment. *Child and Youth Care Forum*, *40*(6), 499–519.

Bettmann, J. E., Russell, K. C., & Parry, K. J. (2013). How substance abuse recovery skills, readiness to change, and symptom reduction impact change processes in widerness therapy participants. *Journal of Child and Family Studies*, *22*, 1039–1050.

Bowen, D. J. & Neill, J. T. (2013). A meta-analysis of adventure therapy outcomes and moderators. *The Open Psychology Journal*, *6*, 28–53.

Bowen, D. J. & Neill, J. T. (2015). Effects of the PCYC catalyst outdoor adventure intervention program on youths' life skills, mental health, and delinquent behaviour. *International Journal of Adolescence and Youth*, *21*, 34–55.

Cambridge English Dictionary. (2019). 'Adventure'. Retrieved October 15th 2019 from https://dictionary.cambridge.org/dictionary/english/adventure

Carpenter, C., Cameron, C., Cherednichenko, B., & Townsend, M. (2007). What changes? Marginalised young people's expectations and experiences of a therapeutic adventure in nature. Paper presented at Australian Association for Research in Education Conference, Freemantle, Western Australia.

Carpenter, C. & Harper, N. (2016). Health and wellbeing benefits of outdoor activities. In B. Humberstone, H. Prince, & K. Henderson (Eds.), *Routledge international handbook of outdoor studies* (pp. 59–68). London, England: Routledge.

Crisp, S. (2004). Envisioning the birth of a profession. In S. Banderoff & S. Newes (Eds.), *Coming of age: The evolving field of adventure therapy* (pp. 209–223). Boulder, CO: Association for Experienital Education.

Csikszentmihalyi, M. (1975). *Beyond boredom and anxiety.* San Francisco, CA: Jossey-Bass.

Deane, K. L. & Harré, N. (2014). The youth adventure programming model. *Journal of Research on Adolescence, 24*(2), 293–308.

Dobud, W. (2017). Towards an evidence-informed adventure therapy: Implementing feedback-informed treatment in the field. *Journal of Evidence-informed Social Work, 14*(3), 172–182.

Gabrielsen, L. E., Fernee, C. R., Aasen, G. O., & Eskedal, L. T. (2016). Why randomized trials are challenging within adventure therapy research: Lessons learned in Norway. *Journal of Experiential Education, 39*(1), 5–14.

Gass, M. A., Gillis, H. L., & Russell, K. C. (2012). *Adventure therapy: Theory, research, and practice.* Abingdon, England: Routledge.

Gladwell, V. F., Brown, D. K., Wood, C., Sandercock, G. R., & Barton, J. L. (2013). The great outdoors: How a green exercise environment can benefit all. *Extreme Physiology & Medicine, 2*(1), 3.

Harper, N. J. (2009). The relationship of therapeutic alliance to outcome in wilderness treatment. *Journal of Adventure Education & Outdoor Learning, 9*(1), 45–59.

Harper, N. J., Peeters, L., & Carpenter, C. (2014). Adventure therapy. In R. Black & K. Bricker (Eds.), *Adventure programming and travel for the 21st century* (pp. 221–236). Champaign, IL: Sagamore Venture.

Harper, N., Rose, K., & Segal, D. (2019). *Nature base therapy: A practitioner's guide to working with children, youth and families.* Gabriola Island, Canada: New Society Publishers.

Holman, T. & McAvoy, L. H. (2005). Transferring benefits of participation in an integrated wilderness adventure program to daily life. *Journal of Experiential Education, 27*(3), 322–325.

Hopkins, D. & Putnam, R. (2013). Personal growth through adventure. Abingdon, England: Routledge.

International Adventure Therapy [IAT]. (2019a). *What is international adventure therapy?* Downloaded from the international adventure therapy website August 2019. https://internationaladventuretherapy.org/what-is-iat/

International Adventure Therapy [IAT]. (2019b). *IAT networks.* Downloaded from the international adventure therapy website October 2019. Retrieved from https://internationaladventuretherapy.org/iat-organisations/

Jackson, A. (2016). Childhood neglect: Beyond trauma theory - mechanisms of harm and hope for recovery. Conference poster. Berry Street Childhood Institute.

Jordan, M. & Marshall, H. (2010). Taking counselling and psychotherapy outside: Destruction or enrichment of the therapeutic frame? *European Journal of Psychotherapy & Counselling, 12*(4), 345–359.

Kezelman, C. & Stavropoulos, P. (2019). *Practice guidelines for clinical treatment of complex trauma*. Milsons Point, Australia: Blue Knot Foundation.

Knowles, B. (2013). Journeys in the bush. *International Journal of Narrative Therapy & Community Work, 3*, 39–48.

Loynes, C. (2002) The generative paradigm. *Journal of Adventure Education and Outdoor Learning, 2*(2), 113–205.

Martin, P. & Priest. S. (1986). Understanding the adventure experience. *Journal of Adventure Education, 3*(1), 18–21.

Mitten, D. (1994). Ethical considerations in adventure therapy: A feminist critique. *Women & Therapy, 15*(3–4), 55–84.

Mortlock, C. (1987). *The adventure alternative*. Cumbria, England: Cicerone Press.

Mutz, M. & Müller, J. (2016). Mental health benefits of outdoor adventures: Results from two pilot studies. *Journal of Adolescence, 49*, 105–114.

Norton, C. L., Tucker, A. R., Farnham, M., Borroel, F., & Pelletier, A. (2017). Family enrichment adventure therapy: A mixed methods study examining the impact of trauma-informed adventure therapy on children and families affected by abuse. *Journal of Child and Adolescent Trauma, 12*(1), 85–95.

Norton, C. L., Wisner, B. L., Krugh, M., & Penn, A. (2014). Helping youth transition into an alternative residential school setting: Exploring the effects of a wilderness orientation program on youth purpose and identity complexity. *Child and Adolescent Social Work Journal, 31*(5), 475–493.

Perry, B. D. (2006). Applying principles of neurodevelopment to clinical work with maltreated and traumatised children. In N. Boyd Webb (Ed.), *Working with traumatised youth in child welfare* (pp. 27–52). New York, NY: Guildford Press.

Prochaska, J. O. & DiClemente, C. C. (1982). Transtheoretical therapy: Toward a more integrative model of change. *Psychotherapy: Theory, Research and Practice, 19*(3), 276–288.

Pryor, A. (2009). Wild adventures in wellbeing: Foundations, features and wellbeing impacts of Australian outdoor adventure interventions (OAI). Unpublished doctoral thesis, Deakin University School of Health and Social Development. Burwood, Victoria, Australia.

Pryor, A. (2015). Towards a profession? A question of paradigms. In C. Norton, C. Carpenter, & A. Pryor (Eds.), *Adventure therapy around the globe: International perspectives and diverse approaches* (pp. 572–594). Champaign, IL: Common Ground Publishing.

Pryor, A., Carpenter, C., & Townsend, M. (2005). Outdoor education and bush adventure therapy: A socio-ecological approach to health and wellbeing. *Journal of Outdoor and Environmental Education, 9*(1), 3–13.

Pryor, A., Conway, J., & Pryor, R. (2019). *Human nature adventure therapy - Recre8 program: Evaluation full report*. Whitfield, Australia: Adventure Works Australia Ltd.

Pryor, A., Pryor, R., & Carpenter, C. (2018). *A formative evaluation of the Gippsland wilderness program*. Richmond, Australia: Berry Street Victoria Inc.

Pryor, A., Pryor, R., & Carpenter, C. (2018). *Outdoor adventure interventions – Young people and adversity: A literature review*. Richmond, Australia: Berry Street Victoria Inc.

Quin, B. (1990). The Essence of adventure. In J. Miles & S. Priest (Eds.), *Adventure education* (pp. 145–148). Champaign, IL: Sagamore Venture.

Rae, P. & Nichols, V. (2015). The Aboriginal outdoor recreation program: Connection with country, culture family and community. In C. Norton, C. Carpenter, & A. Pryor (Eds.), *Adventure therapy around the globe: International perspectives and diverse approaches* (pp. 181–194). Champaign, IL: Common Ground Publishing.

Rakar-Szabo, N., Steele, E. J., Smith, A., & Pryor, A. (2019). Regenerate evaluation: Executive summary. Unpublished Research Report, Adventure Works Australia Inc.

Ringer, M. (2003). Adventure therapy: A description. In K. Richards & K. Smith (Eds.), *Therapy within adventure: Proceedings of the Second International Adventure Therapy Conference* (pp. 19–20). Augsburg, Germany: Zeil Verlag.

Ritchie, S., Wabano, M. J., Beardy, J., Curran, J., Orkin, A., Vanderburgh, D., ... & Young, N. L. (2015). Community based participatory research and realist evaluation: Complimentary approaches for Aboriginal health and adventure therapy. In C. Norton, C. Carpenter, & A. Pryor (Eds.), *Adventure therapy around the globe: International perspectives and diverse approaches* (pp. 646–669). Champaign, IL: Common Ground Publishing,

Russell, K. C. (2003). A nation-wide survey of outdoor behavioural healthcare programs for adolescents with problem behaviour. *Journal of Experiential Education*, 25(3), 322–331.

Simpson, D.P. (Ed.). (1991). *Cassell's Latin Dictionary*. London, England: Cassell Publishers Ltd.

Tucker, A., Norton, C. L., DeMille, S. M., & Hobson, J. (2016). The impact of wilderness therapy: Utilizing an integrated care approach. *Journal of Experiential Education*, 39(1), 15–30.

West, S. & Crompton, J. (2001). Programs that work: A review of the impact of adventure programs on at-risk youth. *Journal of Park and Recreation Administration*, 19(2), 113–140.

White, J.T. & Oxon, D.D. (1893). *Latin-English and English-Latin dictionary for the use of junior students*. Harlow, England: Longmans, Green & Co.

Chapter 8

Nature-Based Therapy

David Segal, Nevin J. Harper, and Kathryn Rose

Introduction

As articulated throughout this book, being outdoors can carry with it significant benefits to therapeutic practice. While numerous expressions of this reality are shared, this chapter focuses on the practical application of taking an office-based practice into local greenspaces, parks, and nearby-nature settings. While additional training and skill development may be required for some practitioners to adopt nature-based therapy, this approach is mostly free of technical equipment or specialized knowledge. That said, an ethical therapy practice includes an intentional and informed approach to therapy, which in this case is primarily focused on being in, and in relationship with, nature.

'Nature-based' is the easiest way to locate this practice—by our physical location—often in nearby nature—for therapy in contrast with being indoors or office-based (Harper, Rose, & Segal, 2019). While conventional therapy indoors is envisioned as counselor and client sitting knee to knee or side by side in a quiet and private office, nature-based is simply as it sounds—outdoors, in natural settings. This approach engages a space and place orientation. Both space (where we are at physically) and place (what that space creates in terms of setting, context, activity, feel, etc.) are malleable concepts. We can design sessions based on locations and create conditions or 'environments' we think best fit clients' needs based on assessment and learning through relationship. Both client and practitioner relationships with nature are considered along with the aims for the session and these can be arrived at mutually. It may be that a favorite cove on the beach on an early summer morning is chosen. This setting may provide resources to the client in their developing relationship with nature. Soft early light, cool saltwater breeze, and a preferred log to sit on can be chosen for a session. These variables have been developed through exploration and dialog on what works best for the clients. These are not resources simply for human use or consumption; these are relationships, now established between client and nature, counselor and nature, and the therapeutic relationship exists in the axis between the three, where nature is co-therapist. This healing partnership is an ecological position and can be viewed as a service to our collective health and well-being and to bring us all more in tune with our biological and earthly selves (Berger & McLeod, 2006).

Nature-based therapy is not for every client, family, or even practitioner. This approach is not a panacea, and it is by no means new (see Levy, 1950). We recognize and acknowledge the truth that we are all nature, nature is everywhere, and that nature is a troublesome word to define and work with as a construct. Nature-based therapy was chosen, however, as the best expression of the work we do. We also acknowledge that we are privileged to work and live in traditional and often unceded and contested Indigenous territories. We express this openly, and, participate in efforts to 'decolonize' these lands through our words and actions. That said, while we are doing human reconnection work with nature, we are not suggesting the use of Indigenous cosmologies, or appropriating cultural practices. This relational nature-based work has, however, been informed by cross-cultural traditional ways of knowing where awareness of the interconnection and respect for the earth and her creatures are valued ideas. Robin Wall Kimmerer (Citizen Potawatomi Nation), a SUNY biology professor, speaks about the notion of human-nature kinships (Kimmerer, 2013). Rather than viewing organisms as 'its' or objects, they are instead seen as relatives, embedded in the same web of life as humans and all beings, including the animals, the birds, the mountains, and sky. Nature today, by many definitions, is unfortunately seen as other than human. The modern Western depiction of human-nature relationship is the antithesis of our understanding and approach to healing. Last, we also recognize that connecting children and their families to nature is not a universal approach to health, healing and well-being and acknowledge the limitations of this approach across cultures, social locations, and populations (Harper, Gabrielsen, & Carpenter, 2018).

Key elements of this approach will be briefly described herein: the practitioner's relationship with nature; nature as co-therapist; full body engagement, play and risk; restoration and regulation; and bonding and belonging (see Harper et al., 2019). This chapter will conclude with a case vignette to illustrate the practical application of these elements.

Discussion of Practice

Practitioner's Relationship with Nature

As highlighted above, nature-based therapy's primary concern is repairing the disconnection that has transpired between humans' and their larger ecological self, the biophysical world. As in all meaningful relationships, one needs to be present and attentive in order for the relationship to thrive. In partnering with the natural world to support the healing of others, the clinician should ideally first cultivate and deepen their own relationship with nature (Burns, 2018; Cohen, 1993). This personal practice of connection lays the foundation for all that follows, and they will be able to step into a session ready to receive the gifts from their co-facilitator—the natural world. This is an experiential mode of practice, as described in Chapter 2, and thus the practitioner must experience the interventions themselves before offering them to clients in order to understand the risks, benefits, and significant potential for meaning and change they offer. Whether it be a consistent practice of sitting and observing nature, building one's own skills in sensory awareness, outdoor survival, and knowledge of local plants/animals, or just spending time exploring the local landscape.

Further, the suggestion of activities and sharing inspiring stories from one's own nature connection practices can be done with authenticity as the practitioner is drawing from their lived experience, not something they have read or heard from a third party. Most importantly, nature-based therapy is intended to be more than a theory, technique, or tool. Nature is being accessed as a valuable teacher and the intention is ideally a reciprocal healing exchange. The transformative power is in the strength of the relationship and this begins with the practitioner's own recognition of their larger ecological self. On a nervous system level, if a practitioner shows up in a regulated state, with their own social engagement system activated due to their connection with the natural world, this can create a poignant therapeutic context for a client to step into. On a practical level, when a counsellor has developed both comfort and knowledge of the local geography, ecosystems, flora, fauna, and both Indigenous and non-Indigenous history/culture of the place, they will have a richer contextual awareness and thus more avenues to draw on to assist in developing their clients' connection.

Nature as Co-therapist

Accepting nature as co-therapist is a central component of nature-based therapy. Introducing this three-way relationship between client, therapist, and nature to the counselling literature, Berger and Mcleod (2006) suggested cultivating nature as an active partner in the healing process. The concept of drawing on nature for healing of mind, body, spirit, and community is certainly not new. Examples of cultures where world and self are inextricably connected and where this relationship forms the center of healing practices has been evident in many land-based cultures' way of life for millennia (see Chapter 5, for example). In the context of nature-based therapy, the focus is on strengthening the clients' relationship with nature without falling into traps of viewing nature as something separate to be used for personal gain. Developing a sense of reverence and respect toward nature, an ongoing recognition for our inextricable embeddedness, and a sensitivity to the ways dominant co-lonial narratives and practices may be operating out of awareness are essential in collaborating with nature (Jones & Segal, 2018). Harper et al. (2019) adopted Joseph Cornell's (1989) four stage 'flow learning' approach to connecting with nature; (1) awakening enthusiasm, (2) fo-cusing attention, (3) direct experience, and (4) sharing inspiration. In each of the stages, personal nature-connection can be enhanced, and opportunities for nature to be a co-facilitator arise and are worthy of further exploration for their function in therapy.

At the beginning of each outdoor session, nature is able to assist in the therapeutic process by awakening a sense of vitality, aliveness, and pres-ent moment awareness. For people who already have a strong ecological identity, this can be facilitated by providing an opportunity to recon-nect through silence and gratitude. For those who are less connected, introducing playful experiences which ground and cultivate presence are ideal. This 'awakening of enthusiasm' (stage 1) sets the tone for the type of receptivity that is required to fully embrace the experiences to come.

Focusing attention (stage 2) affords endless possibilities for discov-ery and psychological and emotional benefits, through tapping into sen-sory awareness. By focusing awareness on one's outer landscape, this allows for the development of observation skills that underpin many of the self-awareness and tracking of internal experiences that follow. By directing one's attention to the myriad ways nature is expressing her-self, clients are given an opportunity to practice being in their 'observ-ing self'—a beneficial mind state which is a cornerstone of mindfulness practices and third wave cognitive behavioral therapy models such as acceptance and commitment therapy (Hayes, 2019).

In the third stage, Cornell (1989) talks about having direct experi-ences (stage 3) with nature which are enhanced by the presence of awe, wonder and sensory awareness. A key element is to be client-centered and allow for wandering and unstructured explorations to unfold. Fur-ther, cultivating a culture of awareness and appreciation for stillness allows for nature to be centered in the experience and her subsequent mysteries and stories to emerge more readily. By allowing nature to act as co-therapist, the practitioner can remain present and be ready to lend a hand when needed and encourage further engagement by asking ques-tions or reflecting what they are seeing unfold.

Another avenue worth exploring are opportunities to develop out-door living skills. Learning the basics of fire making, shelter building or wild foraging allows clients to interact directly with nature while de-veloping a sense of self-efficacy and enhanced capability to take care of some of their basic needs for food, shelter, and warmth. When pursuing this path, it is essential that the practitioner have sufficient training and knowledge to ensure safe and respectful practice and lessons.

Tuning into the metaphoric possibilities of nature is encouraged due to the valuable enhancement of self-awareness and learning that is possible. While metaphor can assist clients young and old to express the seemingly ineffable, or elucidate concepts such as impermanence or life cycles, it is important to note that when metaphors are imposed, they may actually shut down exploration and learning. Hence the importance of allowing metaphors to emerge amidst the unfolding exploration versus imposing them on the situation or misaligning them with how the client is interpreting the experience.

In Cornell's (1989) final stage, sharing inspiration (stage 4), participants pass along meaningful stories of their nature connection. Being in nature and having rich experiences is essential but not sufficient on its own to meet the aims of enhancing health and nature connection, or meeting client's therapeutic needs. Offering space to share stories, be heard, and present to others adds another dimension to the experience. Specifically, (1) stories of connection help to narrate oneself as belonging to the web of life, versus isolated and alone, (2) personal stories of growth and development are able to be witnessed by a caring community (in group or family sessions) and become more solidified in their life, and (3) telling the stories of our connection with nature shifts us out of dominant ethnocentric and individualized notions of reality and opens possibilities for other cultural stories to be possible. The process of re-authoring, witnessing and challenging dominant discourses are common practices adopted from narrative therapy (Madigan, 2019).

Full Body Engagement, Play, and Risk

Experiential learning and play can be engaging and assist in building rapport between client and therapist and also connection between client and family members. Play is a combination of our social engagement and sympathetic arousal systems, which is a healing state (Stanley, 2016) as it allows a person to learn how to regulate their arousal levels. Co-regulation is available through play and allows for further practice of social and emotional skills which can then be beneficial in other settings. The intentional stimulation of the social engagement system, a branch of the autonomic nervous system, is an intervention growing in interest with practitioners and researchers alike (Kain & Terrell, 2018). Play, risk, and full-body engagement allows for clients to access a range of psychological and nervous system states in a safe manner. Learning to navigate risks, for example, affords a state of being that is present-moment focused, and develops resilience which is highly needed in our safety conscious society (see Chapter 11 for more on sensory integration).

Restoration and Regulation

The incidence of mood disorders in North American youth such as anxiety and depression, and the prevalence of ADHD diagnosis continue to rise (Merikangas et al., 2010). The capacity for children to effectively manage social skills and emotional regulation in schools is declining so much so that even kindergarten teachers are overwhelmed with the high needs in their classrooms. It is obvious to us that the nervous systems of our children and youth are dysregulated, and both children, parents and teachers need more tools. As can be seen from the research, time spent in nature has a powerful effect on restoring attention, relaxation, and heart rate (Mygind et al., 2019). In essence, nature is an effective co-regulator for the nervous system—it can serve to down regulate a hyperaroused nervous system (someone who is anxious, angry, stressed) and it can up-regulate a hypoaroused nervous system (those who are depressed, low energy, withdrawn). Nature has this effect because of how it can restore attention, with soft and varied visual stimulation, and natural rhythms and cycles (think of waves lapping the shore), and the potential for movement, curiosity, and exploration that nature invites (Kain & Terrell, 2018). When we bring children out into nature, we can support the stimulation of their ventral vagal nerve (the nerve which supports the social engagement system and puts a break on the sympathetic fight/flight response) through connecting them to their environment, and inviting movement, connection, and awareness. Furthermore, through inviting the child/youth to play in nature within a therapeutic context, we are pairing the social engagement system with the sympathetic system which helps to teach the child how to regulate and stay in connection with others while in a state of heightened adrenaline/cortisol (excitement and nervousness). Thus, the next time the child is in the school yard playing a game, and gets frustrated, they may have developed a higher tolerance for discomfort, and more capacity to pause and redirect their energy in positive ways.

Bonding and Belonging

At its core, nature-based therapy is a systems approach to healing—one that directly addresses the client's relationship with self, family, community, and the wider web of life in which they live. Moving beyond talking about these relationships, this approach explores these relationships intimately and experientially through meeting the child/youth out in the local parks and wild spaces that they call home, often including their family members in the process. Through meeting with youth on a regular basis in these spaces, they develop a sense of bonding and belonging with the local flora and fauna, witnessing it through seasonal changes, through the emergent wildflowers or the wilting leaves. Nature is able to become what John Bowlby (1973) describes as a stronger, wiser other, setting the seeds for a consistent and available resource in their life which they can easily access and which does not judge.

An emphasis is placed on the importance of working toward healing the whole family system when working with children and youth, and nature-based therapy offers a rich setting for engaging the whole family. Getting outside of the office walls, allows for a breaking down of barriers and intimidation from 'expert' and 'problem,' to a sense of play, exploration, shared curiosity, and teamwork/collaboration. The possibility of having experiences of positive connection through the inspiration that the natural world offers means that we can work directly on healing attachment wounds through corrective experiences, on reducing family stress, and practicing new ways of relating. Nature-based therapy can engage a wide variety of interventions in the outdoors—from simple running/hiding games, to teamwork initiatives, to trust activities, to sensory awareness and shared wonderment and attunement to the diversity of life. For many families, whose days are patterned with high stress, conflict, labels, and barriers, the opportunity to experience play, joy, laughter, openness, and trust with one another is invaluable.

Theory, Research, and Efficacy

Nature-based therapy has been found in the literature as a treatment for mental health issues, stress, depression, anxiety, learning difficulties, and pain management for more than a decade now (Berger & McLeod, 2006; Corazon, Stigsdotter, Jensen, & Nilsson, 2010; Grahn & Stigsdotter, 2010). Numerous definitions and descriptions of practice can be found making the task of sharing the theory, research, and outcomes of nature-based therapy as difficult at best. What follows, however, is a brief review of research outcomes and expressions of theory supporting nature-based therapy.

Hospitals, sanatoria, monasteries, and treatment centers through the centuries have been built in beautiful natural settings for a reason. As Stigsdotter et al. (2011) stated:

> There are therefore long held beliefs that human health and well-being are influenced positively by spending time in natural settings. Gardens, pastoral landscapes and natural environments with small lakes and meadows are depicted as places where people can be

restored both mentally and physically. Beneficial properties are attributed to activities in nature, where one experiences natural daylight, fresh air and greenery.

(p. 312)

The activities available to patients or clients in these settings often included walks in nature, gardening, physical exercise, and the consumption of nutritious food often grown on site. It is easy to consider the holistic nature of these settings and services in that they address the patient from most, if not all aspects of their physical, mental, cognitive, and spiritual selves (Stigsdotter et al., 2011).

Annerstedt and Währborg (2011) systematically analyzed the literature on what they defined as nature-assisted therapies in an effort to identify nature's contribution to public health services. Finding 38 sources of controlled and observational studies, the researchers looked at participant characteristics, type of intervention, and study qualities. Overall, they concluded that a "small but reliable evidence bas supports the effectiveness and appropriateness of these approaches as a relevant resource for public health" (p. 371). Of interest to this text on outdoor therapies is the authors inclusion/exclusion criteria and search terms upon which their study was designed. Search terms included *wilderness*, *garden*, *nature-based*, *ecotherapy*, *adventure*, or *green care* reflecting other chapter titles. While practices may be long-standing, the definitions, and practice similarities and differences are still emerging in the literature and fields of service.

Specifically, Annerstedt and Währborg (2011) found more rigorous studies (i.e. high quality) to be a bit ambiguous as to positive outcomes, although stating that the findings were generally favorable. Studies in the low to moderate quality range overwhelmingly showed positive health improvements. Studies traversed a wide range of populations and included nature-assisted interventions for substance use, stress, ageing, somatic disorders, developmental disabilities, psychiatric disorders, attachment, and behavioral disorders. The researchers pointed out that their review was inclusive of a broad range of interventions and thereby makes conclusions harder to put forth. They also called for further research to support human-nature therapy in general, stating, "even though quite a lot of research has been reported on the association between human health and environment, only a few have been defined in a strict therapeutic or intervention pattern" (p. 383).

Corazon, Schilhab and Stigsdotter (2011) put forth theoretical ideas relating to nature-based therapy regarding the relationship between bodily involvement and cognition. The authors drew upon neuroscience to argue that "explicit learning is actively supported by bodily involvement with the environment" (p. 161). The authors shared that sensory-motor systems of the body are engaged through variety of terrains, weather, and types of activities, suggesting a dynamic and holistic modality. The following case vignette illustrates some of the key principles and the possibilities of nature-based therapy.

Case Vignette

A common occurrence is for families to seek out nature-based counselling following several trials with office-based modalities. They hope an alternate approach may meet the unique needs and disposition of their child. In one instance, Miriam, a ten-year-old struggling with debilitating worry, stomach aches, trouble falling asleep, and feelings of overwhelm and panic occurring at school, agreed to try a nature-based approach. Her mother had noticed she was much happier and calmer when playing outside and she was intrigued by the idea that counselling could occur in a space she loved so much. Her early years included her parents separating, which was really hard on the family. Currently, her dad was living in another city with almost no contact. Further, she recently started at a new middle school and this change had overwhelmed her capacity to cope, resulting in the need to seek out counselling.

Prior to the first session, the counsellor held an intake meeting with both mom and daughter which included discussing presenting problems, family history and existing connection with nature (ecological assessment), and to share what was involved in nature-based therapy. It was agreed that Miriam and her mom would attend together to learn how to better manage anxiety, as well as provide opportunities for them to have reparative experiences. Miriam's anxiety had resulted in increased conflict with her mother, such as getting to school in the morning or going to sleep at night, which understandably had taken its toll on their relationship and exacerbated her symptoms.

The sessions began with nature-based play and exploring the local forested park. The mother was encouraged to follow her daughters' lead, bringing forth curiosity and her own child-like self. Sessions would start with an experiential check-in involving moving between two trees and placing themselves where they believed they were at in response to questions such as, how are you doing in this particular moment, the past week, at school/work and other relevant areas. The therapist encouraged naming current feelings, without judgment and deepening these accounts. They were also invited to say what they were grateful for in the forest that day (awakening enthusiasm). Additionally, the concept of sensory awareness was emphasized, and a short-guided mindfulness exercises would prompt them to notice different colors and shades of greenery, listen to the forest sounds, and feel the various textures such as the wind on their face, warmth of the sun, or softness of the moss. These exercises would assist in shifting their focus from the busyness of their day and into the present moment (directed attention). A combination of hiding and sneaking games and also client-led wandering and exploring were offered during the first few sessions.

Near the end of the session, everyone would be given an opportunity to notice their 'inner landscape' and name what they were feeling and thinking after their forest adventure (sharing inspiration). These initial sessions, although they did not explicitly address the presenting concerns just yet, had a number of important aspects. First, it allowed for a strong therapeutic alliance to be established between the family and the counsellor, as well as between the family and nature (bonding and belonging). Further, Miriam and her mother experienced opportunities for reparative connection which was a relief from the constant strain and opposition that was occurring at home, serving to fill up their connectivity bank. These first few sessions also started to build skills of awareness by inviting opportunities to immerse themselves in their outer landscape and then transferring those skills to their inner landscape of feelings, thoughts, and sensations.

On one of those early meetings the weather was quite rainy and despite the wetness, Miriam was engaged in her explorations of a determined slug making its way across the trail. This experience allowed for a number of metaphors to arise. First the ways in which emotions are like the weather. How they shift and change, how we do not have control over them, but how we can adjust how we relate to them (nature as mentor). Also, the determination of the slug was likened to the same tenacity Miriam was showing in her relationship with anxiety and how she continuously works hard to figure out ways to stay at school and tolerate the uncomfortable sensations and negative thoughts (Nature as mirror). In these specific instances, little time was spent exploring these metaphors, as the priority was to encourage an immersive experience in the forest, however the discovery of the slug and the ways Miriam navigated the rain was brought back in later sessions during conversations specifically about anxiety. The rationale was to first work on regulation and the development of awareness skills. After which, parts of sessions were spent specifically exploring how anxiety is showing up in their lives and how they are managing. Also, they learned from the local animals, such as watching the way ground birds reacted to people walking by, and noticing how the birds' nervous systems were responding effectively to keep them safe.

These experiences allowed for discussions about Miriam's nervous system and how she too has an alarm system, which has been alerting her to danger at school and at night. It was possible to use the analogy of the birds to explain how if they stayed in their nest and never took risks, they would not be able to get food and survive. To extend the metaphor, invitations to go on adventures and look for challenges that she could overcome, such as crossing logs and climbing trees were offered during the sessions. During the challenges, the counsellor would model the challenge and self-regulating behavior by verbalizing their inner experience, such as "I know this is scary, and part of me wants to stop, but I also know I can do this." They would also provide examples of self-regulating behavior such as taking big deep breaths, and naming feelings, or asking for assistance. Subsequently, Miriam would be given an opportunity to navigate the challenge with the support of the therapist and her mom. Over time, she was developing the skills to face the uncomfortable feelings associated with anxiety, learning how to name her feelings and sensations, as well as developing the confidence to take action in the presence of fear. She was motivated to challenge herself and she understood that avoidance would continue to contribute to anxiety having control over her life. Thus, she was willing to bring these skills and confidence into her classroom and at nighttime. Importantly, these efforts were further supported by her mom's presence. Miriam's mom was developing both a conceptual and felt experience of nature connection practices as well as learning ways she can support Miriam with co-regulation, and awareness skills, and attuning to her needs.

Finally, each session would end by offering memorable or favorite experiences (shared inspiration), reflections on the progress that was being made, and relevant teachings from the plants and animals, could be discussed. In this context, the nature-based approach allowed for visceral, lived experiences of regulation and modeling that may not have been as readily available for Miriam and her mother within an office setting. It also provided opportunities for enhanced connection and gratitude between mother and daughter.

Conclusion

The rationale, elements of practice, and research base for nature-based therapy has been described in the hopes that interested practitioners can conceptualize partnering with nature as co-therapist in a meaningful way. It has been suggested that enhancing clients' connection with nature allows for reciprocal benefits for individual, familial, and planetary well-being. A case vignette was offered to help elucidate the practice of nature-based therapy in the context of a child struggling with anxiety and the art and science of the approach has hopefully become more clear. Although nature-based therapy is by no means new, the field is beginning to articulate the interventions, skills and practices required to help clients enhance their connection and make positive and lasting change.

References

Annerstedt, M. & Währborg, P. (2011). Nature-assisted therapy: Systematic review of controlled and observational studies. *Scandinavian Journal of Public Health, 39*(4), 371–388.

Berger, R. & McLeod, J. (2006). Incorporating nature into therapy: A framework for practice. *Journal of Systemic Therapies, 25*(2), 80–94.

Bowlby, J. (1973). *Attachment and loss: Separation* (Vol. 2). New York, NY: Basic Books.

Burns, G. W. (2018). *Nature guided therapy: Brief integrative strategies for health and wellbeing.* London, England: Taylor & Francis.

Cohen, M. J. (1993). Integrated ecology: The process of counseling with nature. *The Humanistic Psychologist, 21*(3), 277–295.

Corazon, S. S., Schilhab, T. S., & Stigsdotter, U. K. (2011). Developing the therapeutic potential of embodied cognition and metaphors in nature-based therapy: Lessons from theory to practice. *Journal of Adventure Education & Outdoor Learning, 11*(2), 161–171.

Corazon, S. S., Stigsdotter, U. K., Jensen, A. G. C., & Nilsson, K. (2010). Development of the nature-based therapy concept for patients with stress-related illness at the Danish healing forest garden Nacadia. *Journal of Therapeutic Horticulture, 20,* 33–51.

Cornell, J. B. (1989). *Sharing nature with children II: A sequel to the classic parents' & teachers' nature awareness guidebook.* Nevada City, CA: Dawn Publications.

Grahn, P. & Stigsdotter, U. K. (2010). The relation between perceived sensory dimensions of urban green space and stress restoration. *Landscape and Urban Planning, 94*(3–4), 264–275.

Harper, N., Rose, K., & Segal, D. (2019). *Nature-based therapy for children, youth and families.* Gabriola Island, Canada: New Society Publishers.

Harper, N. J., Gabrielsen, L. E., & Carpenter, C. (2018). A cross-cultural exploration of 'wild' in wilderness therapy: Canada, Norway and Australia. *Journal of Adventure Education and Outdoor Learning, 18*(2), 148–164.

Hayes, S. (2019). *A liberated mind: How to pivot towards what matters.* New York, NY: Avery.

Jones, A. T., & Segal, D. S. (2018). Unsettling ecopsychology: Addressing settler colonialism in ecopsychology practice. *Ecopsychology, 10*(3), 127–136.

Kain, K. L. & Terrell, S. J. (2018). *Nurturing resilience.* Berkeley, CA: North Atlantic Books.

Kimmerer, R. (2013). *Braiding sweetgrass: Indigenous wisdom, scientific knowledge and the teachings of plants.* Minneapolis, MN: Milkweed Editions.

Levy, M. M. (1950). Outdoor group therapy with preadolescent boys. *Psychiatry, 13*(3), 333–347.

Madigan, S. (2019). *Narrative therapy* (2nd ed.). Washington, DC: American Psychological Association.

Merikangas, K. R., He, J. P., Burstein, M., Swanson, S. A., Avenevoli, S., Cui, L., ..., & Swendsen, J. (2010). Lifetime prevalence of mental disorders in US adolescents: Results from the National Comorbidity Survey Replication–Adolescent Supplement (NCS-A). *Journal of the American Academy of Child & Adolescent Psychiatry, 49*(10), 980–989.

Mygind, L., Kjeldsted, E., Hartmeyer, R. D., Mygind, E., Bølling, M., & Bentsen, P. (2019). Immersive nature-experiences as health promotion interventions for healthy, vulnerable, and sick populations? A systematic review and appraisal of controlled studies. *Frontiers in Psychology, 10*, 943.

Stanley, S. (2016). *Relational and body-centered practices for healing trauma: Lifting the burdens of the past.* New York, NY: Routledge.

Stigsdotter, U. K., Palsdottir, A. M., Burls, A., Chermaz, A., Ferrini, F., & Grahn, P. (2011). Nature-based therapeutic interventions. In K. Nilsson, M. Sangster, C. Gallis, T. Hartig, S. De Vries, K. Seeland, & J. Schipperijn (Eds.), *Forests, trees, and human health* (pp. 309–342). Dordrecht, Netherlands: Springer.

Chapter 9

Equine and Animal-Assisted Therapies

Heather White and Kay Scott

Introduction

The idea of incorporating an animal into psychotherapy sessions can be an intriguing option for mental health professionals exploring ways to engage clients in meaningful inner-self exploration, processing, and discovery (Brooks, 2006). Horses and dogs, for example, commonly participate in animal-assisted therapies (Hartwig & Smelser, 2018). This chapter will share theories underpinning equine and animal-assisted therapies, highlight research outcomes, and discuss the professional ethics and guidelines to consider relative to one's scope of practice. When it comes to providing psychotherapy services incorporating animals, a thorough understanding of the other species we are bringing into our work is paramount, and the timeless adage of "do no harm" extends to the animals we choose to partner with in addition to our clients.

Cultural and Historical Perspectives

Animals have been present in human society's construction, first through the concept of animism: the belief that all living beings have a spirit or soul which is heavily influenced by the external environment which could bring forth good fortune or misfortune. In classical times and the *Age of Enlightenment*, animal relationships were further refined in the human psyche as symbolic of certain values or traits, and with this, bringing the notion that animals were less feared and more revered for the qualities they possessed. Ultimately, human-animal relationships and companionship has shaped the development of human culture (Serpell, 2010).

One of the first references involving animals in therapy comes from the 1600s when John Locke discussed incorporating animals to help children develop a sense of empathy (Chandler, 2012; Fine, 2010 as cited in Compitus, 2019). The first written account of the use of animal-assisted interventions in health care was in the 1790s at York Retreat in England (Hines, 2003). Animal-assisted therapy was first utilized in a hospital setting at St. Elizabeth's in Washington, DC around 1919 where dogs were part of the therapeutic recreation for psychiatry patients (Barker & Barker, 2019). Even the father of modern psychotherapy, Sigmund Freud, included his dog Jofi in his work with patients (Shubert, 2012). In the United States, Boris Levinson brought attention to the modality when he brought his dog Jingles into his work practicing child therapy in the early 1960s (Levinson & Mallon, 1997).

According to Crossman (2017), animal-assisted interventions are used across a variety of settings, such as counseling centers, court houses, prisons, airports, universities, psychiatric facilities, sites of natural and human-caused disasters, and in corporate offices. They are used to reduce stress and improve well-being, across many cultures and genders.

Three elements associated with incorporating animals in psychotherapy include professional competency, human and animal welfare, and ethical obligations (Fine, 2010). Involving animals in psychotherapy settings looks to the larger areas of species-specific welfare, training, and animal husbandry considerations when creating and implementing practices. A spotlight remains centered on an ecological perspective, highlighting the interconnectedness of all living things. In this work, specific therapeutic skills are enhanced by knowing how to effectively incorporate animal-assisted therapy skills with tradition counseling and mental health treatment skills (Stewart, Chang, & Rice, 2013). It would be easy to assume that the desire to interact with the animal will make the therapeutic practice easier. However, including animals in psychotherapy can elicit significant emotional responses and clinicians need to remain aware that these interactions serve to enhance clinical work, rather than simply being thought of as the work itself (Ekholm-Fry, 2013).

Philosophical and Ethical Issues

The philosophical underpinnings in the field of animal-assisted interactions are guided by the professional disciplines, such as social work, psychology, or counselling, of the individual(s) facilitating the interaction as well as animal welfare practices which continue to develop. Additionally, what differentiates approaches within the animal-assisted therapies may be dependent on the population an individual is working with.

The Delta Society was integral in the formation of the field of animal-assisted interactions (Hines, 2003), providing definitions and guidelines for the inclusion of animals in human health settings. Since then other organizations have created reports and guidelines surrounding competencies and guidelines for the inclusion of animals in human helping professions (Jegatheesan et al., 2014–2018; Winkle, Dickson, & Simpson, 2019). For example, the American Counseling Association was the first professional mental health membership body to develop such competencies, which included practitioners having awareness about the potential limitations of human-animal interactions in therapy and using effective judgment for determining the impact of an animal on a counselling session (Stewart, Chang, Parker, & Grubbs, 2016).

Research involving animal sentience is growing, showing both an increased need for additional studies focused on positive emotional states of animals as well as bolstering animal welfare as an integral aspect of our interactions with animals (Proctor, Carder, & Cornish, 2013). *Partnering* is a term often used by animal-assisted therapy practitioners of their animal colleague or co-therapist (Scott, 2017). Howie (2015) outlined a "Therapy Dog's Bill of Rights" which highlighted the consideration of power and control dynamics involved in human-animal interactions. Nina Ekholm-Fry (2019) wrote;

> A larger ethical issue in the equine-assisted therapy field not frequently discussed relates to social justice and rights, which are central to mental health fields … The therapeutic environment, which includes therapist, client, horse and environment, cannot be fully therapeutic if the perceived position of power that the therapist has is overlooked, and the same goes for the position of power vis-a-vis the horse. When clients who experience marginalization in their daily lives also sense it in the therapeutic environment, the therapeutic relationship, which, in equine-assisted therapy is expanded to include the horse, is not beneficial.
>
> (p. 130)

Within the area of scope of expertise, animal-assisted therapy has become more formally understood to describe a practitioner acting within their profession's code of ethics, formulating a documented treatment plan and goal(s) for their patient(s)/client(s) with the inclusion of an animal. Ekholm-Fry (2019) stated, "If a therapist is intending to provide equine-assisted therapy … education, training, and supervision is needed for counselors in how to merge their theoretical framework and clinical skills with the nature of equine-assisted therapy and the facilitation thereof" (p. 128).

Theory, Models, and Research

A variety of mental health theories underlie the 'why' of incorporating animals into clinical practice. Two primary theories are Bowlby's (1969) attachment theory and Wilson's (1984) biophilia hypothesis.

Considered by many in the field of animal-assisted therapy to be its theoretical foundation, the biophilia hypothesis, introduced by Edward O. Wilson (1984), proposes that humans are innately imbued to pursue interactions with nature and the natural world, including animals. This internally driven interest in natural surroundings, and 'love of life' has been explored by others since Wilson's original theory (DeLoache, Pickard, & LoBue, 2011; Serpell, 1986).

When it comes to discussions of connectedness, attachment theory is the groundwork for working alongside animal colleagues in therapy. Developed by John Bowlby (1969) and further refined by Mary Ainsworth (1978), attachment theory states that individuals form varied types of relationships with others based upon each their formative relationships and, most influentially, that with the individual's primary caregiver. Attachment theory also extends into ethology via specific behavior and interspecies dynamics.

Animal-assisted interventions have been integrated into mental health work based on a variety of other theoretical perspectives. In Scott's (2017) study, practitioners stated they incorporated animal-assisted therapy into psychodynamic, Rogerian/relational, role theory, social learning theory, and experiential theory. Chandler, Portrie-Bethke, Minton, Fernando, and O'Callaghan (2010) noted their use with Adlerian, behavioral, cognitive-behavioral, existential, gestalt, person-centered, reality, and solution-focused work suggesting interdisciplinary approaches aligned with animal-assisted therapy.

The neurobiological processes involved in interactions between humans and animals continue to be studied to better inform the mechanisms behind its effectiveness. As indicated earlier, the theoretical foundations informing animal-assisted therapy apply not only to the humans involved in these interactions, but to the animals involved as well. Schlote (2019) stated:

> The majority of impacts resulting from trauma and attachment injuries apply not only to humans, but also other mammals, including equines. Species-related differences notwithstanding, overall the impact of adverse experiences shows startlingly familiar and consistent patterns across mammals from a neurobiological, behavioral, and relational standpoint.
>
> (p. 4)

According to Hobfoll et al. (2007), the five essential elements of trauma-informed practice include promoting a sense of safety, calming, a sense of both self-efficacy, and collective efficacy, connectedness, and hope. Safety, physical and psychological, are paramount for animal-assisted therapies and when considering the size differential (big or small) and the inability to communicate with words, animal-assisted approaches rely heavily on all of one's senses to maintain connection and safe practice (Winkle et al., 2019). In discussing how to "congruently communicate" with horses, Vidrine, Owen-Smith, and Faulkner (2002) reminded us of the need to be our authentic selves as we will share "body awareness and intention" with the co-therapist horse (p. 591).

In considering theoretical foundations and rationale for incorporating animals into psychotherapy services, and specifically treatment of trauma, Ekholm-Fry (2019) suggested:

> By utilizing the simultaneously experiential, somatic (mind-body focused), and relational aspects of equine-assisted therapy, therapists can enhance evidence-based trauma treatment in a setting that can be less threatening for many: together with other animals outside the confines of a traditional office.
>
> (p. 128)

In summary, Stewart et al. (2013) found four themes which impact the service provider's approach to animal-assisted therapy in counseling practice. These included (1) the approach requires a unique set of skills and competencies, (2) the providers who deliver the services feel that they have a 'highly developed' working relationship with the therapy animal, (3) inclusion of animals impacts the therapeutic process, and (4) that inclusion of animal-assisted intervention changes the scope of the traditional worker/client relationship.

Unfortunately, like other outdoor therapies, animal-assisted therapy suffers from a lack of clarity on models for practice. This is the central area where professional development and research are needed to move animal-assisted therapies forward professionally; to be tested in and across therapeutic settings to assess what works for whom (Masini, 2010).

Research

One should always look for direction from the available research. In most cases, meta-analyses and systematic reviews are useful for understanding the breadth of knowledge across a specific model of therapy. Animal-assisted therapy now has data at these levels and the results, while largely positive, are mixed, sometimes contradictory and definitely lacking specific population-related outcomes studies (Anestis, Anestis, Zawilinski, Hopkins, & Lilienfeld, 2014). In one meta-analysis, Waite, Hamilton, and O'Brien (2018) found that animal-assisted interventions yield large effects across several medically relevant outcomes in medical populations with problems focused on pain, anxiety, and distress, suggesting the usefulness of incorporating animals in psychotherapy. Nimer and Lundahl's (2007) meta-analysis found that animal-assisted therapy "shows promise as an additive to established interventions and future research should investigate the conditions under which animal-assisted therapy can be most helpful" (p. 225).

Virues-Ortega, Pastyor-Barriuso, Castellote, Poblacion, and de Pedro-Cuesta (2012) reviewed studies specifically related to poor social functioning and found an improvement in social functioning with moderate effects for depression and anxiety. Hoagwood, Acri, Morrissey, and Peth-Pierce's (2017) systematic review of animal-assisted therapies used with youth at-risk for mental health problems found positive effects for the use of equine therapies for autism and canine therapies for childhood traumas. Similarly, Jones, Rice, and Cotton's (2019) review found canine assisted psychotherapy to have a positive impact on primary diagnoses and symptomatology as an adjunct to standard treatments for post-traumatic stress disorder and anxiety. The work led to increased engagement and socialization in the populations as well as reductions in disruptive behaviors. For individuals with Autism Spectrum Disorder, O'Haire's (2013) systematic review found that, despite positive outcomes in social interaction and communication as well as decreases in problem behaviors, there were severe methodological limitations in most of the studies.

Lundqvist, Carlsson, Sjodahl, Theodorsson, and Levin (2017) reviewed healthcare-related literature and identified 18 quantitative studies of dog-assisted therapy deemed at least of moderate methodological quality. Fifteen studies showed some positive effects, but most showed no statistically significant treatment outcomes. The therapies exhibiting the most potential were those focused on the treatment of psychiatric disorders in both young people and adults. It should be noted that the initial literature search for this review included 1,445 studies. However, only 18 met the inclusion criteria for the analysis illustrating a high quantity, but lack of high-quality, scientific work present to support the practice. Throughout the literature on animal-assisted therapy, there are issues with sampling and small sample sizes, codification of the interventions (i.e. the methodology tested), and assessment of outcomes that impact the quality of the data (Kazdin, 2019). The efficacy of animal-assisted interventions was unclear for Charry-Sánchez, Pradilla, and Talero-Gutiérrez (2018) whose recent systematic review included 23 articles and dissertations on the impact of the animal- assisted interventions on depression, dementia, and other conditions in adult populations. While they also stated the quality of studies as low, they did report the results were generally favorable, and that the level of animal interaction held significant influence on outcomes.

Notwithstanding the limitations of scientific rigor, qualitative research has been conducted to build knowledge around people's experiences incorporating animals to psychotherapy. Service providers who incorporate animals into their practice found their work meaningful for the clients. One provider noted, "I begin to see the relationship start to form and notice that relationship transfer over to me in terms of the relationship that my clients feel" (Stewart et al., 2013, p. 340). Another provider noted, "They (dogs) are a social lubricant, it's a conversation starter, it's an icebreaker. It just changes the tone of the office and I think it changes me as a therapist as well" (p. 340).

Participants in Stewart et al.'s (2013) interviews noted that the inclusion of the animal in the therapeutic process provided opportunities for therapeutic touch, higher levels of therapeutic core conditions, and opportunities for practitioners to prevent burnout and increase their own wellness.

Case Vignette

Clara is a 12-year-old female diagnosed with Autism Spectrum Disorder and Generalized Anxiety Disorder. Clara began receiving psychotherapy services with the inclusion of equines to address a growing concern that her mother had with her decreasing social engagement and increasing anxiety. The equine-assisted therapist worked in collaboration with Clara's regular psychotherapist to create a treatment plan with therapeutic goals and objectives which were in line with the services she already received.

The first session was held in an office-based setting which enabled the therapist to assess Clara's ability for communication and engagement in activities with the therapist, as well as allowing Clara to ask questions about the future sessions she would have with the therapist, aiding in establishment of a therapeutic alliance.

During the second session, Clara and the therapist engaged in a herd observation, with the two beginning the session in the office setting then moving to a room where Clara could view the horses. Clara observed the horses, using a paper and pencil to write down her observations and engaged in active conversation with the therapist surrounding questions about what the horses were doing as they interacted with each other. Clara was told about each horse, their names, ages, and information about general preferences, typical behaviors, and unique characteristics as accrued by the therapist from her previous interactions with each horse. At the end of the second session, the therapist asked Clara which equine she wanted to interact with during her next session. Clara chose the pony she had shown more interest in earlier.

For the third session, Clara and the therapist met in the office where the therapist again let Clara know that she would be learning about horse behavior and interacting with the pony she had chosen. The therapist and Clara went through handouts showing body language and stress signals that horses utilize to communicate. During this time, the therapist and Clara talked back and forth about how each horse pictured might be feeling to be in a situation that would cause them to show that behavior and what might help each horse pictured to feel more comfortable. The therapist and Clara also talked about safety around equines, how to approach them and about how she was feeling while discussing these things. Clara replied she had been nervous and excited to touch the pony and she was worried the pony might not like her. The therapist helped Clara to process this information and discussed a plan of action for Clara to make sure she was feeling comfortable and not overwhelmed. The therapist let Clara approach the pony at her own pace, with the therapist moving slowly with relaxed body posture to model for Clara to follow.

As Clara and the therapist approached the pony, they talked about what it was like in this new and unfamiliar situation, what felt comfortable, and if anything did not, how they could remedy that together. As they walked and talked, the pony picked up his head from the grass, still munching on a mouthful of hay, and walked slowly toward the two which made Clara smile and look to the therapist who acknowledged her response. The therapist smiled and asked Clara what she thought the pony was doing when he whinnied. Clara said, "He's saying hello!" and giggled.

As they were talking, the pony decided to walk over toward the therapist and Clara, to which Clara responded by taking a few steps back and slightly hiding behind the therapist. She peeked around to watch the pony approach. The therapist acknowledged this action and asked if Clara was feeling okay with the pony approaching. Clara said, "yes" with a smile and asked the therapist to say "hi" to the pony first. The therapist greeted the pony first verbally by saying hello in a warm tone of voice and then praising the pony and scratching him slowly and lightly on the shoulder with Clara watching close behind. The therapist asked Clara if she was still feeling comfortable and if she was anxious about touching the pony. The therapist noted that Clara could watch if that felt more comfortable. Clara confirmed that this was more comfortable, and the therapist suggested three deep breaths in and out, as a calming strategy, which they did together.

The pony put his head back down and began grazing next to the therapist, which gave the therapist and Clara more time to talk about how Clara was feeling being so close to the pony. She replied that she was excited that she could interact with the pony if she wanted to. The therapist asked Clara to rate her anxiety and how she's feeling right then by giving a thumbs up (feeling good), a thumb horizontal (feeling somewhat anxious), or a thumb down (feeling very anxious) and Clara gave a thumbs up. The therapist then asked Clara what about this situation was helping Clara not feel anxious, but instead excited. Clara responded, "Well, I had seen Toby last week and he seemed pretty calm. We also just talked about how horses talk to each other. Toby was just saying hello, he doesn't seem bothered by us being in here with him." The therapist asked Clara if she wanted to observe Toby grazing for another minute or two at this closer distance and Clara said, "Yes!" The two watched the pony for a few minutes and then walked back toward the office. As they got to the paddock gate and exited the paddock the therapist shut the gate and asked Clara if she wanted to spend the last few minutes at the fence line near the pony talking about this session, which Clara confirmed she did.

The two talked about Clara's experience in this session and the therapist asked Clara if there was anything from the session she could use in her situation of being in a new middle school with new classmates. Clara replied that knowing what she could expect ahead of time helped her with feeling more comfortable. The therapist suggested that Clara could think of more ways to help her feel more comfortable when it comes to the newness of middle school over the next week and then they could start talking about her ideas at the beginning of the next session, which Clara thought was a good idea. The therapist also shared with Clara that at their next session, they would be doing some more interactions with Toby and trying out different ways of getting to know him that would be comfortable for both Clara and Toby.

Discussion

Hartwig and Smelser (2018) identified that about 92% of mental health practitioners they surveyed perceive animal-assisted interventions as a legitimate modality, and 83% would like to use the approach. Only 57% reported an interest in receiving training in the modality and 12% identified they were already trained.

Mental health practitioners looking to incorporate animals into their psychotherapy practices are strongly encouraged to explore the full breadth of the field, seeking university or other professional-based training programs to gain the skills and knowledge needed. New professionals could also explore supervision through experienced professionals, as well as understanding that when incorporating an animal into psychotherapy services, the practitioner is required to have a thorough knowledge of that species' ethology.

There is a clear need to define the models of care to test them at the level of randomized control trials to see if they function at least as well as other modalities (Ambrosi, Zaiontz, Peragine, Sarchi, & Bona, 2019). Like many of the outdoor therapies, there is a real need to assess and align patient symptoms and personality traits with compatible animal-assisted interventions (Buckley, Brough, & Westaway, 2018).

Finally, and most importantly, there is the question of animal welfare. Glenk (2017) noted that few publications deal with the therapy dog's experience of participating in an animal-assisted intervention and almost none identify specific and very real threats to their welfare. Currently there are few clear conclusions on how the well-being of animals is influenced in the delivery of this type of therapy because of the lack of consistent methodology, the recipient and session characteristics, and the methodological limitations of these studies.

The field of animal-assisted therapies continue to evolve at a rapid pace, and professional development, ethical obligations, education, and skill development for practitioners are gaining ground, and the world is taking notice. Together, we can continue to embark on this journey to put our best foot, hoof, and paw forward toward a bright future for all species involved.

References

Ainsworth, M. D. S. (1978). The Bowlby-Ainsworth attachment theory. *Behavioral and Brain Sciences*, *1*(3), 436–438.

Ambrosi, C., Zaiontz, C., Peragine, G., Sarchi, S., & Bona, F. (2019). Randomized controlled study on the effectiveness of animal-assisted therapy on depression, anxiety, and illness perception in institutionalized elderly. *Psychogeriatric*, *19*, 55–64.

Anestis, M. D., Anestis, J. C., Zawilinski, L. L., Hopkins, T. A., & Lilienfeld, S. O. (2014). Equine-related treatments for mental disorders lack empirical support: A systematic review of empirical investigations. *Journal of Clinical Psychology*, *70*(12), 1115–1132.

Barker, S. B., & Barker, R. T. (2019). Animal-assisted interventions in hospitals. In A. H. Fine (Ed.), *Handbook on animal-assisted therapy: Foundations and guidelines for animal assisted interventions* (pp. 329–342). Cambridge, MA: Academic Press.

Bowlby, J. (1969). *Attachment and loss* (Vol. 1). New York, NY: Basic Books.

Brooks, S. M. (2006). Animal-assisted psychotherapy and equine-facilitated psychotherapy. In N. B. Webb (Ed.), *Working with traumatized youth in child welfare* (pp. 196–218). New York, NY: The Guilford Press.

Buckley, R. C., Brough, P., & Westaway, D. (2018). Bringing outdoor therapies into mainstream mental health. *Frontiers in Public Health*, *6*, 1–4.

Chandler, C. K. (2012). *Animal assisted therapy in counseling*. Routledge.

Chandler, C. K., Portrie-Bethke, T. L., Minton, C., Fernando, D. M., & O'Callaghan, D. M. (2010). Matching animal-assisted therapy techniques with intentions with counseling guiding theories. *Journal of Mental Health Counseling*, *32*(4), 354–374. doi:10.17744/mehc.32.4.u721t21740103538

Charry-Sánchez, J. D., Pradilla, I., & Talero-Gutiérrez, C. (2018). Animal-assisted therapy in adults: A systematic review. *Complementary Therapies in Clinical Practice*, *32*, 169–180.

Compitus, K. (2019). Traumatic pet loss and the integration of attachment-based animal-assisted therapy. *Journal of Psychotherapy Integration*, 29(2), 119–131.

Crossman, M. K. (2017). Effects of interactions with animals on human psychological distress. *Journal of Clinical Psychology*, 73(7), 761–784.

DeLoache, J. S., Pickard, M. B., & LoBue, V. (2011). How very young children think about animals. In P. McCardle, S. McCune, J. A. Griffin, & V. Maholmes (Eds.), *How animals affect us: Examining the influence of human-animal interaction on child development and human health* (pp. 85–99). Washington, DC: American Psychological Association.

Ekholm-Fry, N. (2013). Equine-assisted therapy: An overview. In M. Grassberger, R. A., Sherman, O. S. Gileva, C. Kim, & K. Mumcuoglu (Eds.), *Biotherapy – History, principles and practice: A practical guide to the diagnosis and treatment of disease using living organisms* (pp. 255–284). New York, NY: Springer Science + Business Media.

Ekholm-Fry, N. (2019). Equine-assisted therapy for trauma – Accidents. In K. S. Trotter & J. N. Baggerly (Eds.), *Equine-assisted mental health for healing trauma* (pp. 125–139). London, England: Routledge.

Fine, A. H. (2010). *Handbook on animal assisted therapy: Theoretical foundations and guidelines for practice* (3rd ed.). Oxford, England: Academic Press.

Glenk, L. M. (2017). Review: Current perspectives on therapy dog welfare in animal-assisted interventions. *Animals*, 7, 1–17.

Hartwig, E. K. & Smelser, Q. K. (2018). Practitioner perspectives on animal-assisted counseling. *Journal of Mental Health Counseling*, 40(1), 43–57.

Hines, L. M. (2003). Historical perspectives on the human-animal bond. *American Behavioral Scientist*, 47(1), 7–15.

Hoagwood, K. E., Acri, M., Morrissey, M., & Peth-Pierce, R. (2017). Animal assisted therapies for youth with or at risk of mental health problems: A systematic review. *Applied Developmental Science*, 21(1), 1–3.

Hobfoll, S. E., Watson, P., Bell, C. C., Bryant, R. A., Brymer, M. J., Friedman, M. J., …, Maguen, S. (2007). Five essential elements of immediate and mid-term mass trauma intervention: Empirical evidence. *Psychiatry*, 70(4), 283–315.

Howie, A. R. (2015). *Teaming with your therapy dog*. West Layfayette, IN: Purdue University Press.

Jegatheesan, B., Beetz, A., Ormerod, E., Johnson, R., Fine, A., Yamazaki, K., …, & Choi, G. (2014–2018). The IAHAIO definitions for animal assisted intervention and guidelines for wellness of animals involved in AAI. IAHAIO White Paper. Retrieved July 9, 2019 from www.iahaio.org

Jones, M. G., Rice, S. M, & Cotton, S. M. (2019). Incorporating animal-assisted therapy in mental health treatment for adolescents: A systematic review of canine-assisted psychotherapy. *PLOS One*. doi:10.1371/journal.pone.0210761

Kazdin, A. E. (2019). Methodological standards and strategies for establishing the evidence base of animal-assisted interventions. In A. H. Fine (Ed.), *Handbook on animal-assisted therapy: Foundations and guidelines for animal assisted interventions* (pp. 451–463). Cambridge, MA: Academic Press.

Levinson, B. & Mallon, G. (1997). *Pet-oriented child psychotherapy*. Springfield, IL: Charles C. Thomas Publishing.

Lundqvist, M., Carlsson, P., Sjodahl, R., Theodorsson, E., & Levin, L. (2017). Patient benefit of dog-assisted interventions in health care: A systematic review. *BMC Complementary and Alternative Medicine, 17*(1), 1–12.

Masini, A. (2010). Equine-assisted psychotherapy in clinical practice. *Journal of Psychosocial Nursing and Mental Health Services, 48*(10), 30.

Nimer, J. & Lundahl, B. (2007). Animal-assisted therapy: A meta-analysis. *Anthrozoos: A Multi-disciplinary Journal of the Interactions of People and Animals, 20*(3), 225–238.

O'Haire, M. E. (2013). Animal-assisted intervention for autism spectrum disorder: A systematic literature review. *Journal of Autism and Developmental Disorders, 43*, 1606–1622.

Proctor, H. S., Carder, G., & Cornish, A. R. (2013). Searching for animal sentience: A systematic review of the scientific literature. *Animals: An Open Access Journal from MDPI, 3*(3), 882–906.

Schlote, S. (2019). Integrating somatic experiencing and attachment into equine-assisted trauma recovery. In S. K. Trotter & J. N. Baggerly (Eds.), *Equine-assisted mental health for healing trauma* (pp. 3–18). London, England: Routledge.

Scott, S. K. (2017). Walking the dog when talking is too much: Mental health workers' implementation of animal assisted interventions with adult survivors of potentially traumatic events. *Dissertation Abstracts International Section A: Humanities and Social Sciences.* ProQuest Information & Learning. Retrieved June 10, 2020 from https://search-ebscohost-com.avoserv2. library.fordham.edu/login.aspx?direct=true&db=psyh&AN=2017-05709-13 7&site=eds-live

Serpell, J. A. (1986). *In the company of animals.* Oxford, England: Blackwell.

Serpell, J. A. (2010). Animal assisted interventions in historical perspective. In A. H. Fine (Ed.), *Handbook on animal assisted therapy: Theoretical foundations and guidelines for practice,* (3rd ed., pp. 17–32). Oxford, England: Academic Press.

Shubert, J. (2012). Therapy dogs and stress management assistance during disasters. *The Army Medical Department Journal, 2*, 74–78.

Stewart, L. A., Chang, C. Y., Parker, L. K., & Grubbs, N. (2016). *Animal-assisted therapy in counseling competencies.* Alexandria, VA: American Counseling Association, Animal-Assisted Therapy in Mental Health Interest Network.

Stewart, L. A., Chang, C. Y., & Rice, R. (2013). Emergent theory and model of practice in animal-assisted therapy in counseling. *Journal of Creativity in Mental Health, 8*, 329–348.

Vidrine, M., Owen-Smith, P., & Faulkner, P. (2002). Equine-facilitated group psychotherapy: Applications for therapeutic vaulting. *Issues in Mental Health Nursing, 23*(6), 587–603.

Virues-Ortega, J., Pastyor-Barriuso, R., Castellote, J. M., Poblacion, A., & de Pedro-Cuesta, J. (2012). Effect of animal-assisted therapy on the psychological and functional status of elderly populations and patients with psychiatric disorders: A meta-analysis. *Health Psychology Review, 6*(2), 197–221. doi:10.108 0/17437199.2010.534965

Waite, T. C., Hamilton, L., & O'Brien, W. (2018). A meta-analysis of animal assisted interventions targeting pain, anxiety, and distress in medical settings. *Complementary Therapies in Clinical Practice, 33*, 49–55.

Wilson, E. O. (1984). *Biophilia.* Cambridge, MA: Harvard University Press.

Winkle, M., Dickson, C., & Simpson, B. (2019). AAII standards of practice. Animal Assisted Intervention International. Retrieved July 9, 2019 from www.aai-int.org

Chapter 10

Garden and Horticultural Therapies

Rebecca L. Haller

Introduction and Background

Horticulture is the art or practice of garden cultivation and management (Oxford Dictionary, 2019). Horticultural therapy uses gardening as a basis for wide-ranging human services, including physical and psychological rehabilitation, vocational skills development, behavioral healthcare, social development and inclusion, long-term care and hospice, and overall health and wellness. Program sites are similarly broad, ranging from those that take place in rural farm-based locations to those in more clinical settings, such as hospitals and residential treatment centers. Immersion and connection with nature is found in all of these sites and is considered to be one of the foundational benefits of the work, a catalyst for human growth and development (Haller & Kennedy, 2019). Gardening provides a means to engage program participants in motivational, readily available, accessible, and effective outdoor activities. Adaptive and familiar tasks combined with the plant-rich environments aim to foster psychological comfort and social ease, which often results in positive and functional behaviors.

History, Target Populations, and Key Developments

The roots of horticultural therapy began with an awareness of the benefits of gardening for psychiatric patients as illustrated by Friends Hospital (2019), which built a greenhouse for patients in 1879. During World War II, the use of gardening for healthcare branched into physical rehabilitation and services for people with disabilities, with the establishment of rehabilitation hospitals, garden club programs for returning veterans, and schools to teach those with physical or cognitive disabilities (Davis, 1998). Horticultural therapy was subsequently studied at universities in the United States and degrees began to be offered at Michigan State University and Kansas State University in the 1970s (Davis, 1998; Odom, 1973), combining horticulture with psychology and/or occupational therapy.

A growing recognition of the unique and profound benefits of using horticulture as therapy prompted the establishment of the National Council for Therapy and Rehabilitation Through Horticulture in 1973 to promote the use of horticulture for therapy and rehabilitation (Lewis, 1976). The association was later rebranded the American Horticultural Therapy Association. This group devised a system to recognize professionals in the field, and a core curriculum for university degrees and training programs. Further developments have resulted in a system of professional registration based on education in horticulture/plant science, social science, and coursework specific to the practice of horticultural therapy, combined with a supervised internship (Goodyear & Shoemaker, 2012). This model is currently used in various forms in many countries. In the United States, students typically complete university degree programs prior to the study of horticultural therapy and enroll in university-affiliated certificate programs to focus on horticultural therapy to develop skills for the practice and management of programs (Horticultural Therapy Institute, 2020).

Horticulture programs can be found in hospitals, mental health clinics, rehabilitation centers, vocational training centers, schools, prisons, residential care communities for elders, hospices, farms—both rural and urban, in-home care, public gardens, wellness centers, gardens for healthcare support, and many more. The practice sites and populations served continue to diversify and are usually initiated by enterprising individuals in collaboration with new or established healthcare or human service organizations (Malone & Haller, 2019).

Discussion of Practice

Horticultural therapy uses gardening and plant-related activities as an intervention method to promote cognitive, physical, psychological, and/or social benefits (Malone & Haller, 2019; Relf, 1981). Examples of targeted outcomes include recovery from accidents or illness, health improvement or maintenance, vocational skill development, adaptive approaches to tasks, positive mental health, learned coping skills, improved interpersonal relations, stress reduction, increased strength or stamina, improved sense of purpose, and an overall improved wellness or quality of life.

Generally, there are four elements which are central to horticultural therapy: (1) the client served, (2) active cultivation of plants, (3) defined goals and objectives, and (4) a trained horticultural therapist (Haller, 2017). For most, the client has a diagnosis warranting treatment of some type. The term 'treatment' is used broadly here to include services experienced with clinical approaches, as well as community-based or vocational programs. Alternately, the client may not have a diagnosis and may not be in treatment per se, but rather, is someone who self-selects to participate in a wellness program using horticultural therapy.

In horticultural therapy, intervention or treatment methods focus on the *cultivation of plants* and may include many related indoor and outdoor activities. This is a key element that differentiates this practice from the other outdoor therapies presented in this book. Like equine and animal-assisted therapy, discussed in Chapter 9, horticultural therapy involves active care of another living organism as an essential part of the therapy and is a major motivational and engaging aspect of the work (Lewis, 1996). Participants in horticultural therapy programs have identified goals and objectives to which they aspire. These are documented, with progress tracked and recorded to show achievements and outcomes. A trained horticultural therapist possesses clinical and horticultural skills and knowledge, as well as the ability to develop effective programming to maximize positive change in program participants.

Multidisciplinary

Horticultural therapy is a multidisciplinary field, with skills and knowledge needed in the areas of therapy, horticulture, and horticultural therapy (Kuhnert, Shoemaker, & Mattson, 1982; Starling et al., 2014). Therapy skills include treatment planning, counseling, interventions, communication, knowledge of populations served, and motivational techniques, to name a few. Horticulture skills of importance include selecting safe and appropriate plant materials and the use of accessible garden and activity spaces. Horticultural therapy practitioners emphasize program design, session planning, modification and adaptations of tasks, as well as site management.

Treatment Process and Treatment Teams

Treatment planning and implementation use a standard process in all therapies and include assessment, goal identification, intervention plan, intervention, documentation, and termination (Haller, 2017). Horticulture therapists apply a multi-pronged approach to assessment, with varied combinations of pre-placement information, self-reported responses, and observations of the client while engaged in horticultural therapy activities. Goals are written as measurable objectives, and the intervention involving horticulture and gardening is designed to address the objectives (Haller, 2017). The intervention itself involves hands-on horticulture combined with therapeutic methods as needed for success and addressing stated objectives. Progress and behaviors related to the stated objective are documented professionally and communicated to specified individuals. The treatment is terminated upon discharge from care, program completion, or other factors. In many settings, treatment teams are an essential part of the process, and may include a variety of practitioners, as well as the client and their family.

Strengths Based

Horticultural therapy is an adaptive modality. Nearly anyone can be involved in some aspect of horticulture despite cognitive, physical, psychological, or social limitations or challenges. A client with an intellectual disability might transplant seedlings independently with appropriate training, consistency, and perhaps pictorial cues or task sequences. A client experiencing compromised mental health may be able to focus and engage in a garden task that does not seem like therapy. Or, a client with behavioral issues may find solace during time spent gardening while learning new behaviors and relationships in the process. To aid in achieving any of these outcomes, the horticultural therapist focuses on the strengths that each client possesses and helps them to discover their personal resources. The gardener may be able to stay on task and focus despite distractions, discover a safe place to experience a well of pleasure from interacting with plants, or discover their strength and resilience through reflection during their time in the garden.

Rituals, Interventions, and Techniques

Horticultural therapy methods are based on active engagement in gardening and related activities. Typically, clients are involved in some type of plant propagation or care as a way to work toward achievable objectives. Programs may also include a variety of other activities connected to the cultivation of plants. For example, during a session, a group may participate in discussion, group support exercises, planning, garden exploration and observation, or utilizing produce (eating, cooking, floral design, selling produce, etc.). The diverse program types offered in horticultural therapy naturally lead to unique and varied programs that are each tailored to a particular population, setting, and desired outcome.

Horticultural therapists routinely use task analysis as a basis for providing clear and consistent instructions and as a tool to modify or adapt the task, space, conditions, complexity, and instructional methods for individuals and groups. The term 'task' is not necessarily tied to a work attitude or approach and may be presented as an activity for mental health, or leisure, or other purposes as suitable to the program type. The therapist bases modifications or adaptations on the skills of the participants and the treatment objectives. Adaptations might include making the task more accessible to enable full participation, such as using a tool that is safe for young children, removing sharp items from the materials available in secure facilities such as correctional centers or psychiatric hospitals, incorporating written or pictorial step-by-step instructions, working in a quiet area without distractions, gardening from a standing position to increase endurance, or working cooperatively to encourage pro-social behaviors.

A key skill of a horticultural therapist in virtually any type of program is to motivate clients. Several factors inherent in working with plants naturally inspire participation. The garden continually grows and changes, reflects the seasons, focuses on life, offers opportunities to nurture, and provides beauty and food. Intrinsic rewards abound for the client gardener who participates in its creation and care. Engaging the client directly in the development and articulation of goals and objectives also naturally leads to the desire and commitment to work toward them (Haller, 2017). Yet, at times the passion and interest in plants by the therapist must 'carry' the activity and incite participation. For instance, clients may be depressed, taking medications that reduce alertness, have memory loss or dementia, have limited social skills or confidence, or be in physical pain, which in turn may affect engagement. Robust knowledge of the diverse possibilities in horticulture as well as a therapeutic connection to and understanding of the individuals served provide the therapist with many options to motivate participation.

Theory, Research, and Efficacy

Philosophical Underpinnings

Theoretical bases for horticultural therapy's efficacy are as mixed as the practice is varied, yet a few principles are common. It universally offers interactions between people and plants, tapping into the benefits that may be gained through these exchanges. Humans as a species evolved in natural settings, and there is a growing body of evidence that connection with nature is essential for health and well-being (Kellert & Wilson, 1993). According to the theory of *biophilia*, humans have a natural and innate affinity for the natural world and are at risk when they are disconnected from it. While a garden is removed from wild natural environments, and has a definite human influence, nature is ever present. Even in therapy sessions that take place indoors due to adverse weather or medical fragility, close contact with plants brings a connection through the multisensory qualities of plants, responding to the seasons, and experiencing a natural rhythm of life.

Outdoor space which is designed for programming may range from a small area to grow food, to extensive facilities for nursery production, to gardens which emphasize a calm and healing environment (Gallis, 2013). Landscape designs that incorporate elements of safety and security, universal design, physical and emotional comfort, positive distraction, and opportunities for engagement with nature enable users who are in a healthcare setting to access the space and experience stress reduction through connection with nature. Roger Ulrich's (1997) *theory of supportive gardens* describes the potential for stress reduction in the healthcare environment, and recommends providing the user a sense of control, spaces for communal interaction to encourage social support, inspiration to get out of bed and move, and plenty of natural distractions in a plant-rich garden.

Attention restoration theory, proposed by Rachel and Stephen Kaplan, recognizes two types of attention (Kaplan & Kaplan, 1989). Directed attention, such as that common in any complex or difficult task, leads to mental and physical fatigue, and has negative impacts such as irritability, poor judgment, lack of concentration, unhappiness, and difficulty coping. Indirect attention, on the other hand, offers restoration from mental fatigue, and may be experienced in natural environments including gardens. Restoration results when the person experiences four elements in an environment: a feeling of *being away* to an *extent* that has enough scope to offer sources for *fascination* that are *compatible* with their intention at the moment.

Brain neuroplasticity informs horticultural therapy practice, particularly in its application to working with those who have experienced trauma. As the client cares for plants, somatic experiences occur. Combined with the support of the therapist who skillfully applies therapeutic use of self and careful choice of activities, trust and new neural pathways are stimulated to develop (LaRocque, 2019).

While horticultural therapy may provide one-to-one treatment, more often it involves a group of clients. *Group work* encourages goal attainment and provides many benefits to individuals (Yalom, 1995), including opportunities to work on social skills, develop altruism by helping others and caring for plants, and gain a sense of hope from group members.

Outcome Studies

Research in horticultural therapy points to positive change in program participants in diverse areas, including psychological, physical, social, cognitive, and overall well-being. Wichrowski et al. (2004) reported that patients in a cardiac rehabilitation program in the United States showed significantly improved mood states and lower heart rate after a horticultural therapy session, indicating its potential usefulness in reducing stress for those with coronary heart disease. In Korea, a horticultural therapy program reported improvements in interpersonal sensitivity, depression, anxiety, participation, and self-concept of persons with chronic schizophrenia (Son, Um, Kim, Song, & Kwack, 2004). Offenders on probation who worked in community service programs in horticulture improved their self-esteem, knowledge of horticulture and environmental awareness significantly over those who did community service in non-horticultural activities. Perhaps even more impactfully, participants in another horticulture intervention showed lower rates of recidivism (Hale, Marlowe, Mattson, Nicholson, & Dempsey, 2005). The role of horticultural therapy in preventing cognitive decline in patients with Alzheimer's disease was researched by gathering data from tests for impairment, medical records, and reports from dietary, nursing, and therapeutic recreation staff. Those who received horticultural therapy better retained memory abilities, attention span, and well-being (D'Andrea, Batavia, & Sasson, 2007). School children in Taiwan who participated in structured horticulture activities gained relationship skills that include enhanced self-concept and self-satisfaction as well as a better sense of control and achievement (Chen, Lou, Tsai, & Tsai, 2014). They also reported that the sessions helped them to control their emotions and that sharing the activities helped them to make friends and feel happier.

Finding meaning is an important part of a process of healing or recovery, and may ease depression, reduce stress, and lead to greater overall well-being (Haller & Kennedy, 2019). With opportunities to care for plants, clients often report a sense of purpose, a new vocation, a reason to get out of bed, anticipation of the future, and the motivation that stems from being needed.

Gardeners often experience *flow* while working in the garden—a state that allows the person to be so engaged in the activity that time passes unnoticed as self-consciousness and worry disappear (Csikszentmihalyi, 1990). Flow may happen in the garden even while in a group, especially when the activity is carefully matched to the therapy needs and skill level of the gardener. Because horticulture offers such a wide array of activities and ways to approach each client, the skilled therapist is able to encourage flow experiences that are deeply satisfying and intrinsically motivating.

Case Vignettes

The following four cases have been contributed by professional horticultural therapists and illustrate the diverse applications and program types described in this chapter.

Inpatient Mental Health for an Individual Who Has Experienced Trauma (Green Mann, HTR)

A woman living in mental health supportive housing was referred by her social worker to attend weekly one-on-one horticultural therapy sessions. She presented as quiet, observant, and calm, and interacted minimally with fellow residents. She experienced social anxiety, especially around male residents. Her stress reactions included further withdrawal from others. Access to the client's chart and conversations with staff unveiled a complex childhood trauma history affecting her core concepts of self and safety, which led to ongoing dysfunction as an adult. The client showed interest in watering the garden and spent a fair amount of each day outdoors, but remained uncomfortable in groups. Her initial goals included attending the horticultural therapy session regularly, practicing English as a second language, and increasing social interactions.

By mirroring the client's behaviors and working contemplatively side by side on gardening tasks such as seeding, planting, and harvesting food crops, a trusting relationship grew naturally. Being in the garden one-on-one with the therapist allowed her to relax and focus on learning new words and tasks. She noticed that the therapist watched for and deflected other residents from trying to join in or watch her work—events that could heighten her anxiety. The therapist documented each session and communicated with staff to extend her interactions through the week.

The time spent together in the garden led to increased confidence with speaking English, displays of curiosity, a desire to do things well, and enthusiasm about particular gardening tasks. She described her tasks to other staff, received compliments on her beautification projects, shared vegetables, made gifts for her family and staff, and expressed thanks for learning new things and having something "good" to do. Staff noticed the client smiling more often. She occasionally attended the weekly horticultural therapy group session. Recently she stood with arms flung wide and said with a smile that "now her life is the best it's ever been."

Vocational Programming for Adolescents with Disabilities (John Murphy, HTR)

In a vocational application of horticultural therapy, Bullington Gardens partners with the local public-school system to offer BOOST (Bullington Onsite Occupational Student Training). This program dovetails with the Occupational Course of Study for high school students with diversabilities. Students are guided through work experiences for four years with a focus on development of basic job skills and fostering independence. Second year students come to Bullington Gardens weekly to work in the gardens doing routine tasks such as mulching, clearing brush, potting plants in the greenhouse, and mowing the lawn. The program stresses prevocational skills, such as being prepared, staying on task, working together, putting forth effort even if the job is not fun, and doing a good job. Self-confidence is also developed as students feel comfortable and succeed in various tasks.

The highlight of the BOOST program is the annual garden competition between four schools. Students design, grow, and construct a garden within a specific budget. One student with dyslexia, which hinders her ability to read and do math, participated in the competition. Teachers reported that during the previous year she had low self-confidence and did not have an active role in the classroom. She thrived, however, in the creativity of designing the garden for her school and emerged as the leader. With a clear vision, she directed the other four students in its implementation and grew her self-confidence, culminating in the presentation of the garden to more than 100 visitors. She became more outspoken and spoke with confidence, learned new skills, and excelled in performing her job and working with customers.

Vocational Programming in a Farm-based Setting (John Fields)

The client represented is a 34-year-old, nonverbal male, diagnosed with autism spectrum disorder, intermittent explosive disorder, mild/moderate intellectual disability, and attention deficit hyperactive disorder. He has a history of becoming physically aggressive toward property, himself, and others when there is a lack of meaningful activity, structure, and predictability in his daily schedule.

He began goal-oriented, agriculture-based horticultural therapy activities in a closely supervised farm environment in order to provide him with positive engaging routines, and to assist him with meaningful activities geared toward behavior management, as well as vocational training endeavors for future job placement. These interventions were introduced gradually over the course of a six-month growing season. Detailed documentation of progress was kept throughout the process. Sessions began with a maximum of 15 minutes of structured activity and increased as the client's ability to tolerate work in completing program objectives.

The client was provided verbal and visual communication to ensure understanding of expected activities, as well as one-to-one staffing and step by step training in a variety of horticulture related duties. Hand over hand assistance, verbal and visual prompting, and support staff modeling were utilized to help teach gardening and greenhouse skills, such as seeding, watering, transplanting, fertilizing, weeding, and harvesting vegetables. By the end of the six-month period, the client was able to tolerate 120 minutes of continuous work with no significant behavioral outbursts observed and improved his knowledge of vegetable gardening and plant care. Horticultural therapy allowed him to qualify for formalized vocational rehabilitation assessment and training, and eventual employment by the agency as a farm assistant.

Therapeutic Programming in Adult Day Care with an Elder (Pamela Catlin, HTR)

The client began attending a therapeutic-focused horticultural therapy program at an adult day center six months after having a cerebrovascular accident, from which he experienced verbal and cognitive deficits, visual challenges, and mobility impairments. As part of the horticultural therapy program, he participated regularly both indoors and out in the universally designed accessible therapy garden. One day he was observed by the horticultural therapist as he pulled himself out of his wheelchair to stand at a waist-high raised bed. This was the first time he had independently initiated such movement at the day center, with the exception of using the toilet with staff aid. Based on this action and his desire to move out of his wheelchair to stand briefly, his horticultural therapy goal was: *"I want to be able to safely stand and stretch while in the center's garden."* From that time on when in the garden, he would stand at the raised garden bed to plant, water or cultivate, with staff "spotting him" for safety purposes. Though he continued to require the use of a wheelchair in daily life, for a brief amount of time on garden days, he experienced momentary relief from sitting, built stamina, improved balance, learned how to safely transfer from a sitting to a standing position, and received a boost in self-esteem from both the process of standing and engaging with nature - always accompanied by a big smile.

Discussion

Trends

As a developing profession, horticultural therapy continues to define its scope, approach, and practice (Haller et al., 2019). The continuum of the use of horticulture for therapy and human service is applied in many ways, from clinical to holistic and from institutional to community-based programming. The type of people served is similarly diverse, with services targeting a widening client base to include people without medical diagnoses. For example, programs may serve college students or working adults who experience stress, children and adolescents with limited outdoor activity and/or poor nutrition, aging adults who are increasingly isolated, and a variety of other populations who benefit from an earth-based therapy that does not feel like therapy. With diversification, leaders in the field have worked to identify the parameters of which approaches fall within the designation of horticultural therapy.

In 2019, the World Health Organization (2019) identified noncommunicable diseases as a major threat to global health. Unhealthy diets and physical inactivity are two of the major risk factors driving this threat—factors which also worsen mental health issues. These factors can be addressed in part by horticultural therapy programs in which participants exercise through active gardening, grow and consume healthy food, and connect those actions to their mental health and well-being. Interest in cultivating food gardens and incorporating them into all types of treatment programs is growing. Stress reduction is also an area of universal application. Even in vocational programming, therapists use garden tasks and environments to reduce stress, leading to positive outcomes. With an increased recognition of the importance of human-nature connection, and the prevalence of gardens in every community, horticultural therapy has many opportunities to have a significant impact on human health in expanding applications.

Implications for Practitioners and Future Research

While a significant amount of research has been done to identify the benefits of experiencing a garden, horticultural therapists regularly observe positive changes in those who actually participate in hands-on horticulture. More research which focuses on the outcomes of active gardening vs. passively being in the presence of plants is needed, as is research which considers the relative merits of a variety of approaches for treatment in horticultural therapy. A limiting factor in conducting quantitative research is that programs offer only small sample sizes and little consistency across programs exists since each program is uniquely tailored to the clients served, the location and program aims. It is hoped that further research will lead to an increased recognition of positive outcomes in the scientific and healthcare communities.

References

Chen, M. L., Lou, S. J., Tsai, W. F., & Tsai, C. C. (2014). A study of the impact of horticultural activities on primary school children's sell-concept, well-being and effectiveness. *Journal of Baltic Science Education, 13*(5), 637–649.

Csikszentmihalyi, M. (1990). *Flow: The psychology of optimal experience.* New York, NY: Harper & Row.

D'Andrea, S. J., Batavia, M., & Sasson, N. (2007). Effect of horticultural therapy on preventing the decline of mental abilities of patients with Alzheimer's Type Dementia. *Journal of Therapeutic Horticulture 18,* 8–17.

Davis, S. (1998). The development of the profession of horticultural therapy. In S. Simson & M. Straus (Eds.), *Horticulture as therapy: Principles and practice* (pp. 3–20). Binghamton, NY: Haworth Press.

Friends Hospital. (2019). History of Friends Hospital, Philadelphia, PA. Retrieved March 5, 2019 from https://friendshospital.com/about-us/our-timeline/

Gallis, C. (2013). *Green care: For human therapy, social innovation, rural economy, and education.* New York, NY: Nova Science Publishers.

Goodyear, N. & Shoemaker, C. (2012). The state of horticultural therapy around the world. *Acta Horticulturae, 954,* 159–189.

Hale, B., Marlowe, G., Mattson, R. H., Nicholson, J. D., & Dempsey, C. A. (2005). A horticultural therapy probation program: Community supervised offenders. *Journal of Therapeutic Horticulture, 16,* 38–49.

Haller, R. (2017). Goals and treatment planning. In R. Haller & C. Capra (Eds.) *Horticulture methods: Connecting people and plants in health care, human services, and therapeutic programs* (2nd ed., pp. 27–36), Boca Raton, FL: CRC Press, Taylor and Francis Group.

Haller, R. L., Kennedy, K. L., & Carpa, C. L. (Eds.). (2019). *The profession and practice of horticulture therapy.* Taylor & Francis Group.

Haller, R. & Kennedy, K. (2019). Horticultural therapy, related people-plant programs, and other therapeutic disciplines, In R. L. Haller, K. L. Kennedy, & C. L. Capra (Eds.), *The profession and practice of horticultural therapy* (pp. 23–44). Boca Raton, FL: CRC Press, Taylor and Francis Group.

Horticultural Therapy Institute. (2020). Horticultural therapy certificate program. Retrieved June 10, 2020 from https://www.htinstitute.org/certificate-program/

Kaplan, R. & Kaplan, S. (1989). *The experience of nature: A psychological perspective.* Cambridge, MA: Cambridge University Press.

Kellert, S. & Wilson, E. O. (1993). *The biophilia hypothesis.* Washington, DC: Island Press.

Kuhnert, K., Shoemaker, J., & Mattson, R. (1982). Job analysis of the horticultural therapy profession. In J. Shoemaker & R. Mattson (Eds.), *Defining horticulture as a therapeutic modality* (pp. 17–38). Manhattan, KS: Kansas State University.

LaRocque, C. (2019). Program example: The interface between horticultural therapy, trauma treatment, and somatic-oriented mental health therapy, In R. L. Haller, K. L. Kennedy, & C. L. Capra (Eds.), *The profession and practice of horticultural therapy* (p. 132). Boca Raton, FL: CRC Press, Taylor and Francis Group.

Lewis, C. (1976). *Fourth annual meeting of the national council of therapy and rehabilitation through horticulture,* September 6, Philadelphia, PA.

Lewis, C. A. (1996). *Green nature/human nature: The meaning of plants in our lives.* University of Illinois Press.

Malone, K. & Haller, R. (2019). Development of the profession. In R. L. Haller, K. L. Kennedy, & C. L. Capra (Eds.), *The profession and practice of horticultural therapy* (pp. 23–44). Boca Raton, FL: CRC Press, Taylor and Francis Group.

Odom, R. (1973). Horticulture therapy: A new education program. *HortScience, 8*(6), 458–460.

Oxford Dictionary. (2019). Horticulture. Retrieved June 10, 2020 from https://www.lexico.com/en/definition/horticulture

Relf, D. (1981). Dynamics of horticultural therapy. *Rehabilitation Literature*, 42, 147–150.

Son, K. C., Um, S. J., Kim, S. Y., Song, J. E., & Kwack, H. R. (2004). Effect of horticultural therapy on the changes of self-esteem and sociality of individuals with chronic schizophrenia. *Acta Horticulturae, 639*, 185–191.

Starling, L., Waliczek, T., Haller, R., Brown, B., Malone, R., & Mitrione, S. (2014). Job task analysis survey for the horticultural therapy profession. *Horticulture Technology, 24*(6), 645–654.

Ulrich, R. S. (1997). A theory of supportive design for healthcare facilities. *Journal of Healthcare Design: Proceedings from the Symposium on Healthcare Design, 9*, 3.

Wichrowski, M., Whiteson, J., Haas, F., Mola, A., & Rey, M. (2004). The effects of horticultural therapy on mood and heart rate in patients participating in an inpatient cardiopulmonary rehabilitation program. *Journal of Cardiopulmonary Rehabilitation, 25*(5), 270–274.

World Health Organization. (2019). Ten threats to global health. Retrieved June 10, 2020 from https://www.who.int/emergencies/ten-threats-to-global-health-in-2019

Yalom, I. (1995). *Theory and practice of group psychotherapy.* New York, NY: Harper Press.

Chapter 11

Nature, Sensory Integration, and Pediatric Occupational Therapy

Kaya Lyons

Introduction

Every day we participate in activities and tasks to help us feel a sense of safety, survival, achievement, growth, and accomplishment. For some, this can be challenged due to developmental delays, injury, trauma, and/ or an accident or illness (Case-Smith & Bryan, 1999). When these obstacles prevent people from completing important daily tasks and participating in meaningful activities, their sense of security and feelings of empowerment are challenged. It is at this stage, that an occupational therapist may be recommended.

The roots of occupational therapy lie in supporting humans to have the functional capacity to participate in daily routines and to develop and maintain a sense of self-worth (Kielhofner, 2009). Occupational therapy is "a client-centered health profession concerned with promoting health and well-being through occupational performance. The primary goal of occupational therapy is to enable people to participate in the activities of everyday life" (World Federation of Occupational Therapists Council, 2019, para. 1).

Occupational therapy practice is extremely diverse and supports people across the life span. Where approaches vary, the key concept of a holistic approach remains consistent throughout occupational therapy practice. This holistic approach considers an individual's relationships (attachment, friendships, family networks, professional supports), environment (physical, emotional, cultural, socio-economic), as well as the foundational skills which underpin function (mental and physical abilities) (World Federation of Occupational Therapists Council, 2019).

Individuals and their families are integral to the intervention process. They aid in establishing goals which are meaningful and unique to the needs and desires of the individual. Cultural beliefs and values are also considered in client-centered goals (Whiteford & Wright St-Clair, 2002). The individual's goals could be using tools to garden, getting oneself dressed, writing, attending school, getting to sleep, walking and navigating around the shops, or catching public transport.

Due to the diversity within the field of occupational therapy, there are a range of therapists that specialize in different areas (injury rehabilitation, child developmental issues, etc.). This chapter focuses on the framework of a pediatric occupational therapist specializing in sensory integration with a trauma-informed approach while incorporating adventure and outdoor settings (May-Benson, 2016).

Challenges with sensory integration affect many people with disabilities and trauma (Baranek, David, Poe, Stone, & Watson, 2006; Ben-Sasson et al., 2007). Sensory integration is the neurological process that organizes sensation from one's own body and from the environment and makes it possible to use the body effectively within the environment (Ayres & Robbins, 2018). Trauma can interrupt and/or disorganize sensory integration. Currently, trauma is defined as singular or cumulative experiences that result in adverse effects on functioning and mental, physical, emotional, or spiritual well-being (Substance Abuse and Mental Health Services Administration, 2018).

When supporting clients with a sensory integration and trauma-informed response, engagement with nature deserves consideration. Being outdoors in nature provides enriched sensory experiences across all sensory systems (Ramshini et al., 2018). Further, many cultural and spiritual rituals lie deeply entwined with nature and nature can be beneficial when considering intervention strategies to support the mental, emotional, and physical needs of individuals (Li et al., 2019). See Chapters 5 and 13 for further detail on this front. Herein lies fertile ground for occupational therapists to provide a sensory integration approach in nature.

Sensory Processing

Humans have eight primary senses: five provide information regarding our environment (touch, smell, sight, hearing, and taste) and the remaining three senses provide information about our body (proprioception—body sensing/locating in space, vestibular—head movement, and interoception—internal states) (Star Institute for Sensory Processing Disorder, 2018). Feeling safe within one's environment stems from the processing and organization of the *external* senses. Feeling secure within one's body comes from the processing and organization of the *internal* senses. It is the relationship between the two, the environment and the body, that provides a platform for individuals to integrate their internal and external senses. If our sensory processing is adaptive, we will feel secure within ourselves, and be available to explore and learn within our environment.

Sensory processing takes place in the lower, primal areas of the brain (the brain stem and limbic system) (Bundy, Lane, Murray, & Fisher, 2002). Processing occurs very rapidly, without cognition. Every millisecond the brain continues to receive new sensory input, integrate the input, and organize adaptive responses. It is no wonder that sensory processing occurs without cognitive thought. If we were more conscious of it, we would find ourselves becoming overwhelmed, tired, or it could even cause shutdown.

Humans are hard-wired to survive as a priority with such processing occurring in our primal brain. As such, an individual's perception of threat, identified through sensory processing, will determine their response (van der Kolk, 2014). If threat is perceived, individuals will act before thinking as a means of surviving. A person may run from a situation when they perceive a loud sound; sometimes before turning to see what the sound was.

Sensory processing integrates with emotional memories and responses within the primal brain; impacting not only what we feel, but how we respond (Davidson & Begley, 2012). Over time an individual's emotional regulation and the perception of self can also be impacted (Davidson & Begley, 2012).

When sensory processing is impacted, our perception of the environment and our body often does not match the situation. An individual may have difficulties with social, emotional, and learning aspects of life (Star Institute for Sensory Processing Disorder, 2018). For example, a person struggling with sensory processing may have difficulty forming and maintaining friendships, sharing and interpreting emotions, appear clumsy, impulsive, have poor self-worth, present with anxiety, and/or aggressive or other behavioral responses. Challenges with sensory processing can occur in isolation, in relation to an associated diagnosis (including autism spectrum disorder, attention deficit disorder), as well as in response to an attachment and/or childhood trauma (van der Kolk, 2014). With such a significant impact on life, the sensory integrative approach might be beneficial for people with such concerns (Bundy et al., 2002).

Trauma

Trauma places additional stress on an individual's system leading to physiological shifts in the body and mind (van der Kolk, 2014). When a person's safety and security is under threat, responses can shift to survival and remain active across daily tasks. As such, responses to sensory input during daily activities become based on a perception of need for safety and defense rather than thriving and connecting. In such circumstances, a trauma-informed, sensory integrative approach might be worth implementing.

A trauma-informed approach to therapy can be utilized alongside a strengths-based framework that is responsive to the effects of trauma (Bateman, Henderson, & Kezelman, 2013). A strength-based focus looks to empower individuals by recognizing and utilizing their strengths to support development, growth, and coping skills, rather than focusing on pathology (Bateman et al., 2013). This trauma-informed approach also highlights the importance of the physiological, emotional, and psychological safety of both the client and the therapist to help rebuild a sense of control and empowerment.

Discussion of Practice

The core principle to a sensory integration intervention is to provide specific sensory input in a way that an individual spontaneously forms adaptive responses that integrate the input (Ayres & Robbins, 2018). It is a bottom-up approach where, considering the individual's responses to sensory input, hypotheses are made regarding an individual's neurological processing within the primal brain. Therapists utilizing a sensory integrative approach aim to identify and understand individual's behaviors as responses. Rather than treating or stopping unwanted behaviors through reward or punishment, for example, therapists implement techniques to support and build the individual's own internal resources (Greenspan & Salmon, 1995).

A sensory integration intervention is commonly provided in a sensory gym clinic, at school, or in the home environment with individuals or groups (Zimmer & Desch, 2012). In these environments, games and activities aim to provide specific sensory input, integrated with emotional responses and thinking as well as attentive tasks. The foundation of the activities is specific to the individual, goal-directed, and the therapist takes the individual's lead to support meaningful function (Ayres & Robbins, 2018).

The therapeutic activities aim to organize the nervous system so that skills can be generalized into the individual's daily life activities. Therapeutic techniques can include the use of: swings; balance/climbing equipment; visual targets; balls, bats and targets; resistance bands; exercise balls; weighted equipment and inclines; specific modulated music; changes of positions of movement; firm pressure therapy brushes; blow toys for breath activation; cause and effect resources; and problem solving activities such as obstacles. The activities support individual's strengths whilst stimulating them, using just the right amount of challenge to develop their emerging skills required for organization and function. Therapy is embedded in the purposeful role of play for children and in meaningful work/leisure/self-care/rest activities for both children and adults (Wilkinson et al., 2019).

Sensory Integration and Natural Environments

Clinical reasoning demands an exploration of the most effective therapeutic interventions and techniques for each individual and the environment(s) within which such therapy could occur (Bennett & Bennett, 2001).

Environments where the nervous system can calm from perceived threat and where an individual can feel connected are ideal; where the client feels safe and secure and the therapist and environment can support emotional connection and confidence. It is here, that we look to understand the inter-weaving of sensory integration therapy, a trauma-informed approach, and outdoor natural environments.

Interaction with the environment is helpful in developing the brain. Through experience and exploration, the brain will organize itself if provided with opportunities (Ayres & Robbins, 2018). Given that the theoretical framework of such an approach is so integrated with the environment, there are vast opportunities for using the outdoors as part of the approach. At this time, however, the integration of such approaches, is not frequently practiced with such specific intention. The value of using nature for sensory integrative therapy is significant and requires further exploration (Harper, Rose, & Segal, 2019).

When considering the properties of nature, the opportunities for sensory integrative therapy are endless. Nature is enriched with opportunities to explore sensory inputs that are often calming to the nervous system due to their balanced nature, and thus encourages individuals to explore and learn. Nature is a place where opportunities for risk, challenge, success, exploration, problem solving, and achievement of new skills comes in vast supply. There is the chance to explore hidden spaces, scale rocks, play in the breaking waves, track animals, read the sun, feel the different textures of leaves, bark, and earth, etc. These activities allow individuals to sense, move, emotionally feel, and connect. These foundations underlie health and well-being (van der Kolk, 2014).

Theory, Research, and Efficacy

Adventure therapy, as discussed in Chapter 7, is commonly defined as "the prescriptive use of adventure experiences, often conducted in natural settings that kinesthetically engage clients on cognitive, affective, and behavioral levels" (Gass, Gillis, & Russell, 2012, p. 1). When considering the sensory, emotional, and cognitive elements to adventure activities, one can begin to weave this into a trauma-informed, sensory integrative approach.

Where such an integrative approach is in its infancy, its empirical base in research is also lacking although my practice experience has demonstrated meaningful change. For example, therapy outcomes include:

- a child being able to go with their family on a bike ride or on a daily outing without having a melt-down;
- a child going on a school camp and staying there the entire time;
- a child returning to school;

- a child forming friendships and playing with their friends;
- a child being able to swim, walk, and swing;
- a family being able to have dinner together, or go on a family trip;
- a teenager indicating their self-worth.

When looking at the impact intervention has on function, current literature supports the relationship between difficulties processing and integrating sensations and performing basic 'activities of daily living' and 'instrumental activities of daily living,' such as sleeping, dressing, eating, engaging in play, and participating in leisure and school-related activities (Chien, Rodger, Copley, Branjerdporn, & Taggart, 2016; Kuhaneck & Britner, 2013; Mazurek & Petroski, 2015). There is also evidence that Ayres' sensory integration therapy improves functional skills and goal attainment (Schaaf et al., 2015; Schaaf, Dumont, Arbesman, & May-Benson, 2017).

The research suggests that sensory integration therapy contributes to successful achievement of an individual's goals, improved well-being, increased motivation to participate in daily tasks, reduced behavioral responses, and improved emotional, motor, play, and sleep development (Cohn, Miller, & Tickle-Degnen, 2000; Cohn, 2001; Pfeiffer, May-Benson, & Bodison, 2018). However, research is limited regarding the use of nature to achieve therapeutic benefits of sensory-integration and a trauma-informed approach.

Interventions for childhood trauma recovery are in their infancy. Recent neurobiological research has suggested complex childhood trauma experiences are associated to neuroanatomical brain structures including those supporting self-regulation and arousal (LeBel & Champagne, 2010; van der Kolk, 2014). Many interventions have been separated into mental health, sensory integration, and the body. Recently, however, there has been a shift to integrating the body with mental health approaches to support development (Ogden, Minton, & Pain, 2006). It is becoming more evident that there is much overlap between individuals sensory processing and trauma responses involving emotions and behaviors to support an integrated approach to therapy.

Further, theorists have explored the therapeutic use of self (see Chapter 2). It is thought that being authentic and sharing can support establishing a working alliance built on trust to achieve growth (Dewane, 2006; Edwards & Bess, 1998; Shulman, 2008).

As research continues to expand, it is imperative that all current therapy is completed with a systematic approach including measurable outcomes to assess change. It is equally important that outcome measures are sensitive enough to change and designed for such purposes. Given occupational therapy is goal focused and client-centered, goal measurement scales have commonly been used to identify positive changes in individual's daily performance including social interaction, behavioral responses, self-care, writing, reading, sleeping, and eating; the Goal Attainment Scale (Smith, 1976) and The Canadian Occupational Performance Measure (2019) as examples.

Further research in individual as well as integrative frameworks of sensory integration and taking trauma-informed approaches to the outdoors may be of benefit to continue to guide therapy and provide support for individuals. This requires careful consideration of fidelity and effectiveness of intervention for specific groups of people on larger scale measurements.

Case Vignette

Bec is an 11-year-old girl who lives in foster care. Her early years were spent living with her mother and father who abused drugs and alcohol. Her foster care environment is consistent, loving, and supporting with firm boundaries and expectations. Bec is an extremely athletic and talented young girl who seeks to control situations, frequently taking a role of the organizer. Her diet is self-restricted to a few preferred foods and her bowel movements are irregular. In daily life, she identifies she is always 'fine' and can complete daily routines outside of the home environment with efficiency.

When in the safe environment of home, however, her need to control situations leads to reduced flexibility to listen to other perspectives, a lack of compliance, and increased emotional responses (yelling, slamming doors, not following instructions). When such responses are discussed with her, Bec is unable to articulate her emotions and instead shifts to shutting conversations down indicating that she is 'fine.' Bec's emotional range is very limited, her thinking is linear and there is reduced glee and playfulness in her interactions. When invited to participate in creative, exploratory tasks, Bec reverts to logical, structured task completion rather than enjoying the journey and flexibility of exploring.

Further, Bec's impulse control is limited during emotionally evoking experiences (such as excitement or anger) as well as tasks that include sensory activation that are not anchored in the body (such as using her phone). When her lack of impulse control leads to not following rules at home, her behavioral responses escalate. These responses are a daily occurrence and are impacting her ability to get ready for school, build and sustain friendships, complete homework, engage in mealtimes, and interact with those around her.

As therapists, we begin to unpack Bec's early trauma and the impact this may have had on her attachment and responses. We hypothesize that the lack of responsiveness from her primary caregivers in early childhood has led to emotional suppression and a survival response to logically think through and control tasks.

In early years, the primal brain develops attachment and security through sensory and emotional connections and experiences with a primary caregiver. When this was not available for Bec, her survival strategy was likely to shutdown these areas to reduce the intensity to sense and feel, and instead to use logic, planning, and sequencing to gain function and meet her needs. While these responses are beneficial (adaptive) and important for survival during immediate situations of early development, these responses are now maladaptive in Bec's life.

Over time, such strategies put excessive strain on the left hemisphere of the brain and reduced activation of the right hemisphere of the brain. This is likely to lead to decreased clarity in thinking, stress, and challenges with aspects of resting and digesting. Further, the strategy to reduce sensory and emotional processing for survival has a negative impact on Bec's ability to socially connect. Forming and maintaining important relationships rely on the processing and authentic connection of touch and emotion sharing. As human beings, it is now known there is a link between social connection, physical health, well-being, and happiness (Davidson & Begley, 2012).

Practically for Bec, sensory integrative therapy in nature is about connecting body, mind, and spirit through relationship, sensation, and emotion. This provides a platform of security, a place to explore, build, and form meaning within her experiences. It is not just about connecting in nature. It is about connecting to each individual sense and linking these processing experiences to emotions; authentically sharing these experiences with others. Walking in the woods becomes exploring what Bec can see, smell, hear, feel, and taste. What draws Bec's attention and what does she find interesting? What does Bec notice in her body about her breath, heartbeat, and her overall feeling? Are there any tight areas in her body or areas that feel relaxed, warm, or cool? Does this change? How?

Coupled with sensory integration there is the added element of right brain to right brain connection through authentically sharing sensory and emotional experiences and connecting (Schore, 2009). There is great value in sharing the present moment whilst walking along in the woods, to the smell of the eucalypt leaf when folded, the sight of red sap dripping from a gum tree, to feel your heart pumping as you walk up the steep hill, or your need for breath as the pace increases. Drawing awareness to the processes that occur subconsciously bring to our conscious mind our inner and outer selves. Notice these sensations, pause to process them, and draw awareness to the changes. Spend time reflecting: what sensation in moments were pleasant, enjoyed, disliked, or not noticed? Share individual perceptions without comparison or judgment, instead curiosity.

It is by connecting the sensory input and emotional experiences in present moments that we may help to develop resources. Resources which Bec now draws upon in her daily experiences, providing a platform of positive memories for sensing and feeling emotions. Building new neurological connections of safety and security. As such, shifting the coping responses from shutdown and suppress, to sense and feel. Bec can now notice when her heartrate is increasing. She can draw awareness to her breath. She is aware that snuggling under a warm blanket helps her to feel calm. Bec enjoys creating with clay and uses this as a way of releasing emotions. Her shifts provide room for her to feel motivated to engage in learning, complete home demands, and begin to build friendships.

Engaging in therapeutic sensory experiences in a natural setting supports opportunities that include calming inputs which evoke positive emotional responses. Current demands of daily life draw awareness away from a sense of self and toward the large, somewhat overstimulating sensory inputs of our technology-based world. Therapy completed in such an environment may limit opportunities to sense and feel organizing input. Being present in natural environments can provide plentiful opportunities to stimulate and strengthen adaptive neurological pathways that organize the primal brain.

Conclusion

There is a wide diversity in the practice of occupational therapy considering the age of individual clients, their diagnoses, and the frameworks in which therapists use to guide an intervention.

As our understanding of sensory integration improves, more individuals are being identified as having difficulties with sensory processing, including those on the autism spectrum and presenting with childhood trauma. There are now many leading professionals across therapeutic fields sharing their knowledge and research regarding how the human body, not just the mind, stores memories which have an impact on health and well-being. These memories influence how a person assumes posture, moves, reacts, explores, learns, and feels. With such an understanding, more therapists are sharing and delivering services which involve sensory integration to support further development of an individual's body, mind, and spirit.

Advancement and use of technology for work, learning, and social connecting brings forth further challenges. Such changes in society place greater stress on individuals' sensory systems. Technology also drives individuals further away from engaging in sensory integrative and nature-based activities. It is here that the biggest challenge for the future lies. Will there be enough therapists driven to provide the services our society needs? Will there be enough quality research completed to advocate the benefits of such intervention for those in need? Will the impact of not participating in such activities be drawn to awareness in communities to aid prevention? Will insurance companies and governing bodies support advancement in such approaches?

At this time of increased knowledge and change, it is important that practitioners continue to share and support one another, to extend frameworks, and complete and publish research. Sensory integrative occupational therapy in nature is a highly specialized field. Where it is important to embrace all those interested in entering the field, it is also very important that support and access to training is made available to ensure that practitioners are qualified and adhere to best practice for the integrity of the field and the safety and interests of those we serve.

References

Ayres, A. J. & Robbins, J. (2018). *Sensory integration and the child*. Los Angeles, CA: Western Psychological Services.

Baranek, G. T., David, F. J., Poe, M. D., Stone, W. L., & Watson, L. R. (2006). Sensory experience questionnaire: Discriminating sensory features in young children with autism, developmental delays, and typical development. *Journal of Child Psychology and Psychiatry, 47*, 591–601.

Bateman, J., Henderson, C., & Kezelman, C. (2013). *Trauma-informed care and practice: Towards a cultural shift in policy reform across mental health and human services in Australia. A national strategic direction*. Position paper and recommendations of the National Trauma-Informed Care and Practice Advisory Working Group. Lilyfield, Australia: Mental Health Co-ordinating Council.

Bennett, S., & Bennett, J. W. (2001). The process of evidence-based practice in occupational therapy: Informing clinical decisions. *Australian Occupational Therapy Journal, 47*(4), 171–180.

Ben-Sasson, A., Cermak, S. A., Orsmond, G. I., Tager-Flusberg, H., Carter, A. S., Kadlec, M. B., & Dunn, W. (2007). Extreme sensory modulation behaviours in toddlers with autism spectrum disorders. *American Journal of Occupational Therapy, 61*, 584–592.

Bundy, A. C., Lane, S., Murray, E. A., & Fisher, A. G. (2002). *Sensory integration: Theory and practice*. Philadelphia, PA: F. A. Davis.

Case-Smith, J. & Bryan, T. (1999). The effects of occupational therapy with sensory integration emphasis on preschool-age children with autism. *American Journal of Occupational Therapy, 53*(5), 489–497.

Chien, C.-W., Rodger, S., Copley, J., Branjerdporn, G., & Taggart, C. (2016). Sensory processing and its relationship with children's daily life participation. *Physical & Occupational Therapy in Paediatrics, 36*(1), 73–87.

Cohn, E., Miller, L. J., & Tickle-Degnen, L. (2000). Parental hopes for therapy outcomes: Children with sensory modulation disorders. *American Journal of Occupational Therapy, 54*, 36–43.

Cohn, E. S. (2001). Parent perspectives of occupational therapy using a sensory integration approach. *American Journal of Occupational Therapy, 55*, 285–294.

Davidson, R. J. & Begley, S. (2012). *The emotional life of your brain: How its unique patterns affect the way you think, feel, and live and how you can change them.* New York, NY: Hudson Street Press.

Dewane, C. (2006). Use of self: A primer revisited. *Clinical Social Work Journal, 34,* 543–558.

Edwards, J. & Bess, J. (1998). Developing effectiveness in the therapeutic use of self. *Clinical Social Work Journal, 26,* 89–105.

Gass, M. A., Gillis, H. L., & Russell, K. C. (2012). *Adventure therapy: Theory, practice & research.* New York, NY: Routledge.

Greenspan, S. I., & Salmon, J. (1995). *The challenging child: Understanding, raising, and enjoying the five "difficult" types of children.* Reading, MA: Addison-Wesley Publishing Co.

Harper, N. J., Rose, K., & Segal, D. (2019). *Nature-based therapy: A practitioner's guide to working outdoors with children, youth, and families.* Gabriola Island, BC: New Society Publishers.

Kielhofner, G. (2009). *Conceptual foundations of occupational therapy practice.* Philadelphia, PA: FA Davis.

Kuhaneck, M. H. & Britner, P.A. (2013). A preliminary investigation of the relationship between sensory processing and social play in autism spectrum disorder. *OTJR: Occupation, Participation and Health, 33*(3), 159–167.

LeBel, J. & Champagne, T. (2010). Integrating sensory and trauma-informed interventions: A Massachusetts state initiative, part 2. *Mental Health Special Interest Section Quarterly, 33*(2), 1–4.

Li, D., Larsen, L., Yang, Y., Wang, L., Zhai, Y., & Sullivan, W. C. (2019). Exposure to nature for children with autism spectrum disorder: Benefits, caveats, and barriers. *Health & Place, 55,* 71–79.

May-Benson, T. A. (2016). *A sensory integrative intervention perspective to trauma-informed care.* OTA The Koomar Center White Paper. Newton, MA: OTA The Koomar Center.

Mazurek, M. O. & Petroski, G. F. (2015). Sleep problems in children with autism spectrum disorder: Examining the contributions of sensory over-responsivity and anxiety. *Sleep Medicine, 16,* 270–279.

Ogden, P., Minton, K., & Pain, C. (2006). *Trauma and the body.* New York, NY: Norton.

Pfeiffer, B., May-Benson, T. A., & Bodison, S. C. (2018). Guest editorial—State of the science of sensory integration research with children and youth. *American Journal of Occupational Therapy, 72*(1), 1–4.

Ramshini, M., Karimi, H., Zadeh, S. H., Afrooz, G., Razini, H. H., & Shahrokhian, N. (2018). The effect of family-centered nature therapy on the sensory processing of children with autism spectrum. *International Journal of Sport Studies for Health, 1*(4), 1–5.

Schaaf, R. C., Cohn, E. S., Burke, J., Dumont, R., Miller, A., & Mailloux, Z. (2015). Linking sensory factors to participation: Establishing intervention goals with parents for children with autism spectrum disorder. *American Journal of Occupational Therapy, 69*(5), 6905185005.

Schaaf, R. C., Dumont, R. L., Arbesman, M., & May-Benson, T. A. (2017). Efficacy of occupational therapy using Ayres Sensory Integration®: A systematic review. *American Journal of Occupational Therapy, 72,* 1–10.

Schore, A. N. (2009). Right-brain affect regulation. In D. Fosha, D. J. Siegal, & M. Soloman (Eds.), *The healing power of emotion: Affective neuroscience, development, and clinical practice* (pp. 112–144). New York, NY: WW Norton & Company.

Shulman, L. (2008). *The skills of helping individuals, families, groups, and communities* (6th ed.). Belmont, CA: Thomson Brooks/Cole.

Smith, D. L. (1976). Goal Attainment Scaling as an adjunct to counseling. *Journal of Counseling Psychology, 23*(1), 22–27.

Star Institute for Sensory Processing Disorder. (2018). Your 8 senses. Retrieved June 9, 2020 from https://www.spdstar.org/basic/your-8-senses

Substance Abuse and Mental Health Services Administration. (2018). Trauma-informed approach and trauma-specific interventions. Retrieved June 8, 2020 from https://www.samhsa.gov/nctic/trauma-interventions

The Canadian Occupational Performance Measure. (2019). The Canadian occupational performance measure: COPM. Retrieved June 10, 2020 from http://www.thecopm.ca

van der Kolk, B. A. (2014). *The body keeps the score: Brain, mind, and body in the healing of trauma*. New York, NY: Viking.

Whiteford, G. & Wright St-Clair, V. (2002). Being prepared for diversity in practice: Occupational therapy students' perceptions of valuable intercultural learning Experiences. *British Journal of Occupational Therapy, 65*(3), 129–137.

Wilkinson, K., Rossi, J., Scott-Cole, L., Silvia, R., Allman, C., Kennedy, A., ..., & Schutt, K. (2019). Outdoor play in pediatric OT practice. *American Journal of Occupational Therapy, 73*(4-1), 7311515352P1.

World Federation of Occupational Therapists Council. (2019). World federation of occupational therapists: WFOT. Retrieved June 10, 2020 from https://www.wfot.org/about/about-occupational-therapy

Zimmer, M. & Desch, L. (2012). Sensory integration therapies for children with developmental and behavioral disorders. *Pediatrics, 129*(6), 1186–1189.

Chapter 12

Surf Therapy

Jess Ponting

Introduction and Background

Surfing is an Indigenous sport with a long cultural history dating back thousands of years. While surfing reached its pre-colonial zenith in the Hawaiian islands where it was integral to cultural and social life, surfing was also taking place on bundled reed canoes in pre-Incan Chan Chan fishing communities in Peru as early as 300 BC (Warshaw, 2004). Similarly, Atlantic West Africa (Dawson, 2018; Pearson, 1979), Papua New Guinea (O'Brien & Ponting, 2013), Fiji (Ponting & O'Brien, 2013), and islands throughout Polynesia (Crawford & Wright, 1994; Lanagan, 2002) were all host to pre-colonial surfing traditions.

Captain James Cook and his crew onboard the *Resolution* observed a Tahitian man in a dugout canoe riding waves in 1777 and the ship's log noted that Cook "could not help concluding that this man felt the most supreme pleasure while he was driven so fast and smoothly by the sea" (Warshaw, 2004, p. xi). American Calvinist missionaries arrived in Hawaii in 1820 and despite intense negative pressure on surfing from colonial powers and the decimation of the Indigenous Hawaiian population by as much as 95% at the hands of colonial diseases, surfing survived (Walker, 2011). American novelists Jack London and Mark Twain both wrote with breathless enthusiasm about surfing in the first decade of the new century. In parallel, emerging industrialists began to leverage surfing as tourism destination marketing imagery for Hawaii and as a hook for coastal real estate and railway developments in southern California (Ponting, 2017). Indigenous Hawaiian Olympic swimming champion Duke Kohanamoku seeded surfing into Australian culture in 1912 but it was not until the late 1950s that a Hollywood-driven teenage fascination with surfing swept the Western world. Within ten years, surf media and surf apparel industries emerged, went global in the 1980s, and became billion dollar industries at the turn of the 21st century (Ponting, 2017; Warshaw, 2004). Today surfing is a global sport, 106 countries are members of the International Surfing Association, which will oversee the sport's Olympic debut in Japan, 2020. Surfing is practiced by approximately 35 million people around the world (O'Brien & Eddie, 2013) and growing at a rate of 30% per year (World Surf League [WSL], n.d.). The global surf industry has been estimated to be worth between $70 and $130 billion annually (O'Brien & Eddie, 2013).

The earliest reported instance of formalized surf therapy was in 1996 when the non-profit organization *Surfer's Healing* was established in southern California after Israel and Danielle Paskowitz serendipitously discovered the calming effect surfing had on their son Isaiah, who had been diagnosed with Autism Spectrum Disorder (Surfers Healing, n.d.). This was followed in 1998 by Santa Cruz based organization *Ride a Wave* in 1998 (Ride a Wave, n.d.). Established in 2017, the International Surf Therapy Organization (2019) defined surf therapy as "the evidence-based, clinically-guided, and safely delivered use of surfing and play in and around waterways as a therapeutic vehicle in the prevention and treatment of social, behavioral, health, economic, and other challenges" (n.p.). Several aspects set it apart from other nature-based and outdoor therapies. Clients are engaged in an intense sensory experience, quite literally immersed into a dynamic outdoor environment that is constantly moving and changing. This requires equally constant physical responses. Surf therapy yields both moments of quiet reflection and bonding between waves, as well as the thrill and pleasure of riding bands of energy created by the sun.

Surf therapy has expanded beyond its historical roots as an intervention for children with autism (see Cavanaugh & Rademacher, 2014; Stuhl & Porter, 2015) to encompasses children with disabilities other than autism (Armitano, Clapham, Audette, & Lamont, 2015; Clapham, Armitano, Lamont, & Audette, 2014; Moore, Clapham, & Deeney, 2018), foster youth in residential care (Gaspar de Matos et al., 2017), at risk youth (Colpus & Taylor, 2014; Godfrey, Devine-Wright, & Taylor, 2015; Hignett, White, Pahl, Jenkin, & Le Froy, 2017), people suffering addiction (Harris, 2015), terminal illnesses (Nichols, 2014), and combat veterans (Caddick et al., 2015a; Crawford, 2016; Fleischmann et al., 2011; Rogers, Mallinson, & Peppers, 2014). In addition, there are many different therapeutic modalities including one day events, programs that run once per week over a number of weeks, programs that run several days per week over a number of weeks, multi-day or week surf camps with surfing each day, and long term programs that run once per week over many years.

Discussion of Practice

Stuhl and Porter (2015) reviewed three separate programs targeting children with autism through a range of modalities, from two-day camps to six-week and eight-week programs. Their assessment found a considerable amount of support for surf therapy based on the positive results that all the existing research has demonstrated accrues to participants. The outcomes of the three programs suggested that programs targeting children with disabilities, and in particular Autism, should incorporate the following components:

- Social, cooperative, motor, and sensory activities to complement the surfing experience
- Involving families in the overall experience
- Fostering a greater sense of community between participants and between participants' families
- Learning and leveraging the individual learning styles of participants
- Ensuring a participant/staff ratio of at least 1:1
- Teaching specific social skills in surfing and non-surfing activities
- Integrating social learning into other life settings, e.g., school, future camps, possible future roles as mentors or volunteers
- Ensuring participants are free to explore and perform without fear of failure (Stuhl & Porter, 2015, p. 254)

While these components can be integrated to achieve maximally effective outcomes in children with disabilities, they are not directly transferrable to the context of wounded combat veterans. No studies to date have attempted to distill best practice inclusions for the veteran community. In order to understand what practice looks like for this community, the author interviewed the co-founder of the longest running surf clinic for wounded veterans (interview can be heard at https://csr.sdsu.edu/).

Nico Marcolongo is a veteran of two tours of Iraq as a Major in the US Marine Corps and co-founded the Naval Medical Center San Diego Surf Clinic (Surf Clinic). For more than a decade, the Surf Clinic has been running weekly sessions for veteran and active duty military suffering from visible and invisible combat wounds. The Surf Clinic began when individual veterans were put in touch with Major Marcolongo by the San Diego Navel Medical Center and he enlisted a lifeguard to help facilitate surfing experiences for veterans with multiple amputations. The efficacy was immediately obvious and the program grew to become a Department of Defense sanctioned rehabilitation clinic.

Reintegration to civilian society can be a major challenge for wounded veterans (Dustin et al., 2016). The Surf Clinic involves a large group of veterans gathering in a public place, allowing them, perhaps for the first time since their injury, to feel comfortable in a public setting. It can take several visits to the beach for the 'troops' to feel ready to attempt surfing, and several more before they successfully catch a wave, but each stage of this process is increasingly empowering and represents a restoration of control over their lives. Surf therapy has proven particularly helpful for bilateral above the knee amputees who initially struggle with new prostheses. According to Major Marcolongo (personal communication, 2015):

> when they're in the water and they're surfing, they have an advantage. They can pop up on the board, [with their] low center of gravity, and they can pick it up very quickly. That's really exhilarating. They really take to it. You don't have to have limbs to have that mobility in the water. The ocean is a great equalizer for a lot of the injuries.

Marcolongo identified several key elements that contribute to its efficacy in this modality and with this population. First, time spent floating between waves allows the troops to feel the calming, healing power of the ocean, experience wildlife interactions (e.g., dolphins, seals, pelicans), and have time to reflect and process what has happened to them. Second, the adrenaline rush of riding a wave can help satisfy veterans' need for excitement and adrenaline that sometimes leads to destructive behaviors (Caddick et al., 2015b). Third, overcoming the dangers presented by a rough ocean involves learning to calmly surrender to the unpredictability of the ocean. According to Major Marcolongo, learning to be calm in the face of unpredictable challenges leads to healing and directly translates into better outcomes for those struggling to reintegrate to civilian society with physical and psychological challenges. Finally, the act of surfing a wave in the Surf Clinic is an individual challenge while the process of going surfing with the Surf Clinic group is very social. There is constant banter between troops about conditions and wave choice. This discussion acts to build trust in the team. Active duty troops work as a team by carrying out individual tasks that help the team as a whole, so the individual/team dynamic is familiar and reassuring. It helps participants to think beyond themselves and their physical/psychological injuries which, Major Marcolongo says, leads to healing.

Theory, Research, and Efficacy

Ample research has been conducted indicating that experiences in nature, and in particular physical activity in nature, can bestow therapeutic benefits on participants from various populations (Coon et al., 2011; Dustin et al., 2016). Coastal environments have attracted particular attention from researchers coining terms, such as 'blue space' (White et al., 2010), 'blue gym' (Depledge & Bird, 2009), and 'blue mind' (Nichols, 2014) to describe how being around and in water positively influences well-being. Nichols (2014) specifically explored the neuroscience of not just exposure to coastal and marine environments but surfing in particular.

Surfers have long noted the personal benefits they experience from surfing, and scholars have begun to explore this from a number of perspectives. Steven Butts (2001), for example, found that surfing "satisfies a psychological need, one that clears the mind and cleanses the spirit" (p. 1). Surfing has also been positioned as 'high-risk leisure' (Stranger, 1999, 2011). Traditionally high-risk leisure has been lauded for the catharsis it can instigate when juxtaposed against rapid social change (see Giddens, 1991). Pearson (1979), for example, saw surfing as an alternative anchor for identity construction by post World War II youth who felt stifled by outdated modernist expectations. Stranger (1999, 2011), by contrast, found value in the sensual, embodied experiences of thrill and risk. Similarly, Farmer (1992) concluded that thrill generated by risk taking, and often articulated as 'stoke,' was the most important factor in motivating people to surf.

Professor of religion, Bron Taylor (2007) considers surfing to be:

> a profoundly meaningful practice that brings physical, psychological, and spiritual benefits ... a religious form in which a specific sensual practice constitutes its sacred center, and the corresponding experiences are constructed in a way that leads to a belief in nature as powerful, transformative, healing, and sacred.
>
> (p. 923)

Anderson (2013) suggested surfing represents "a means to experience the transcendent" (p. 954) and that surfing spaces are both spaces of spirituality and liminal spaces. The liminality of the surf zone means that it is "not just a place to play, but can also be recognized as a cathedral of the spirit, functioning as an important resource for human happiness, alongside physical and spiritual well-being" (p. 967). Nerothin (2018) found that riding waves, and the intervals between riding waves, are very different experiences that complement the overall impact of surfing on well-being. While wave riding is thrilling and conducive to flow experiences and involves a balance of risk and reward, the intervals between are far more reflective and restorative periods. While quite different, both allow a shift of attention away from everyday mundanities and lead to enhanced short-term wellness in terms of physical health, mental fitness, and emotional well-being (Nerothin, 2018). These types of benefits, which most surfers inherently understand, clearly lend themselves to therapeutic interventions.

The body of outcome research specifically focused on surf therapy is small but growing. Rogers et al. (2014) conducted pretest-posttest examinations of 14 veterans at a post-combat clinic engaged in a five-week program where participants surfed one day each week. The study revealed significant improvements across measures of post-traumatic stress disorder and depression and concluded that surf therapy could serve as a useful intervention of veterans suffering with the disorder. Crawford (2016) conducted quantitative, repeated-measure research across 95 veterans participating in one week residential camps (staying in the same hotel, surfing for three to four hours each day of the week) and determined that there was substantial positive change in the areas of self-efficacy, posttraumatic stress disorder, and reduced depression. However, further research is needed to determine if the impacts last beyond the 30 days. Fleischmann et al. (2011) found surf therapy simultaneously addressed multiple issues including pain, vestibular impairment, and cognitive symptoms by incorporating elements of "hydrotherapy, strength training, balance rehabilitation, and group supportive therapy" (Fleischmann et al., 2011, p. 27).

Caddick et al. (2015a) used a qualitative narrative approach based on interviews and participant observation of 15 combat veterans over the course of 18 twice-weekly camps and a three-week residential program in the United Kingdom. They found that participants experienced almost complete respite from their post-traumatic stress disorder symptoms during their participation. This respite was described as interrupting a 'cycle' of the disorder's symptoms leading to an overall improvement in well-being facilitated by keeping the veterans focused on the present and having an enjoyable experience to both reflect on and look forward to, and facilitating relationships with other veterans that helped combat the loneliness and social isolation that characterize post-traumatic stress disorder.

Another stream of research deals with modalities targeting children with disabilities and special needs. There is significant overlap in the findings of these studies. For example, Moore et al. (2018) conducted interviews with the parents of 13 children with disabilities and behavioral challenges aged between 8 and 19 who participated in an eight week summer program consisting of two one-hour surf sessions per week. Parents reported increased balance, muscle tone, and stamina along with benefits from sensory inputs such as the tightness of the wetsuit and the feel of the crashing waves that manifest as a regulation of negative behaviors (e.g., aggression). In addition, parents reported improved attitude, outlook, and self-confidence, as well as social skills and feelings of inclusion. These benefits were reported to have been transferrable to many other facets of the children's lives. Armitano et al. (2015) alternatively looked only at physical benefits of an eight-week ST intervention consisting of weekly surf sessions for children with disabilities (mostly autism and Down syndrome) and showed measurably improved upper-body strength, core strength, and cardiorespiratory endurance.

The authors also noted observed increases in self-confidence, gains in social development, and decreased anxiety among participants.

Devine-Wright and Godfrey (2018) conducted a longitudinal study of an annual six-week intervention for young people with mental health needs. Participants received a two-hour surf lesson once a week for six weeks. Having run annually since 2013, the program has provided participants with opportunities to remain engaged through additional surfing lessons outside of the program and opportunities to volunteer in the following years' programs. Analysis of five years of data shows that clients experienced an increase in confidence, physical and mental health, and well-being which was sustained over time. Similarly, Hignett et al. (2017) investigated the efficacy of a 12-week program of weekly surf lessons for children aged 12–16 who were excluded, or in danger of being excluded, from mainstream school as a result of behavioral issues. The research concluded that participants' physical fitness increased along with their self-worth, positive social relationships among peers, and pro-social behaviors. Similar results were reported in a study that involved foster youth in residential care in Lisbon, Portugal across an eight session, twice-weekly program (Gaspar de Matos et al., 2017).

The existing literature supports the consensus among researchers that the benefits of surf therapy are real. Further, the benefits appear to have significant overlap across different populations and modalities. Godfrey et al. (2015) outline some of the key components of surf therapy that translate across all of the studies carried out to date (including those published after Godfrey et al.'s work). They include the following: (a) the ocean is a restorative environment; (b) participants feel a spiritual connection with nature; (c) surfing is a highly sensory experience that facilitates learning and develops resilience; (d) participants feel included; (e) being recognized and supported builds positive self-concept and self-esteem; and (f) contact between participants, and between participants and instructors builds trust.

Case Vignette

The following vignette describes the work of many surf therapy organizations that are focused on serving children with, most commonly, autism, Down syndrome, speech disorders, and seizure disorders. Many organizations serving these populations use a modality where surf therapists and clients ride together on large 'tandem' surfboards allowing quick and easy access to the thrill of riding a wave even for those with no previous experience in the ocean. Best Day Foundation has taken this a step further in its development of the 'Surf Chair 2000' which incorporates a modified Formula 1 carbon fiber racing car seat bolted to a very large customized surfboard that enables a surf therapist to stand behind the chair and accommodate clients who are unable to stand (Best Day Foundation, n.d.-a, n.d.-b).

While the details of service delivery and focal points of the experience vary between organizations, most follow a similar trajectory to A Walk on Water who describe the experience they provide to clients, who they refer to as athletes, on their website's FAQ page in the following way:

> From the moment you arrive, our volunteers will welcome you and assist your family with carrying your beach gear, getting you checked-in and making sure your liability waivers have been signed, providing you with special giveaway items, explaining how your day will proceed, getting your athlete fitted into a wetsuit and flotation device, accompanying your athlete while they await their turn, introducing your athlete to their surf therapist, familiarizing your athlete with what to expect in the water, providing the opportunity to surf multiple waves, celebrating your athlete's accomplishment in a group trophy ceremony, providing healthy snacks, lunch and drinks, and offering plenty of high-fives, smiles and positive vibes.
>
> (AWOW, n.d.)

Most organizations highlight the importance of surf therapists and clients spending time together before heading out to sea to establish a level of comfort and familiarity. On entering the water, the first stop is out beyond the breakers to sit and experience nature, feel the calming rhythm of the swell and the warm, full-body sensory experience of the wetsuit. Once the client has found a sense of calm in the moment, the surf therapist then begins catching waves in what are most commonly 30–60 minutes surf sessions, varying by organization, allowing as many as 10 waves to be ridden depending on conditions.

Surfing is inherently risky. Providing surf therapy for children with disabilities amplifies those risks and introduces many more so many organizations exceed that there is one surf therapist per client at all times they are in the water. In addition, staff or volunteers are stationed in the water where the therapy is taking place with the goal of being able to reach clients who require assistance within a few seconds. Finally, staff or volunteers are placed along the beach to carefully observe clients and render assistance as needed (Lambert, 2019).

Many surf therapy organizations go to special lengths to celebrate their clients and create an atmosphere of inclusion that may be lacking from their daily lives. This celebration can take the form of announcements over a public address system set up on the beach, award and trophy ceremonies, and photography and videography celebrating surf therapy experiences that can become cherished items among clients. One parent, quoted in Jones (2017), participating in the 'Special Surfer' program, described the importance of regular surf therapy and the artefacts it produces for her family as follows:

> We don't have school pictures. He's not in school long enough to have them taken. So our house has five-year-old surfer Ben. Six-year-old surfer Ben. Seven-year-old surfer Ben. Every year, our house is littered with pictures of him surfing and the success that he's had. This is the Christmas concert that I never get to go to; this is the Little League practice that we'll never make; this is the Mothers' Day crafts that were never made in school and sent home. This is everything that every parent gets to experience daily that I don't get to experience.
>
> (n.p.)

Surf therapy organizations have reported the value of their services as perceived by the parents of their clients, and these reports seem to mirror the results reported by efficacy studies. The feeling of total acceptance by surf therapists, participants, and their communities during surf therapy sessions are very clearly valued by families. For example, one parent whose child participates in the Best Day Foundation surf therapy reported that:

> Best Day really has been a life-altering experience for my daughter. She has adopted the "I can do anything" attitude, and her whole outlook on life has changed. She also has more confidence and better self-esteem. Best Day gave her a place where she belongs; she feels wanted, needed, and loved. The staff remember her and greet her with joy and happiness that she's there, which is something she doesn't get many other places.
>
> (n.p.)

Positive impacts related to a sense of calm and confidence also appear to be somewhat 'sticky' and spillover into life beyond the surf therapy sessions, at least for a time. A parent from the A Walk on Water program reported that significant changes in demeanor, calmness, and ability to sleep soundly persisted for a week after their son's surfing experience.

> The calm and peace my son felt afterwards was evident in the great school bus rides and great school days for the entire week afterwards which was reported to me by his teacher and bus staff. The calmness of his body and smiles on his face and the enthusiastic head nod YES he gave me when I asked him if he had enjoyed the day with all the surfers said it all, not to mention the restorative nights of peaceful sleep that followed.
>
> (AWOW, 2018, n.p.)

Discussion

Surf therapy appears to be on the rise. The number of organizations and the geographies they represent are growing. The International Surf Therapy Organization (2019) currently lists 31 organizations operating in 13 countries. This is far from an exhaustive listing with the International Surf Therapy Organization being a very new organization that is still working to bring the surf therapy world together. Academic interest in the field is growing, government financed efficacy studies are under way (Michalewicz-Kragh, 2019), and government sanctioned and funded interventions are already happening for various populations in the United States and United Kingdom. The adaptive surfing movement is also gaining traction and velocity with the World Adaptive Championships growing steadily year after year.

Rising in parallel with the growth of surf therapy is the emerging surf park industry. Surf parks are large pools or lagoons fitted with human engineered mechanical systems that create high quality waves for surfing (Roberts & Ponting, 2018). Like surf therapy, the surf park industry is nascent but rapidly gathering momentum. Ad hoc surf therapy sessions have been conducted at most of these existing facilities with anecdotal evidence suggesting they were successful. As such, there does appear to be potential for this emerging industry to broaden access to people who do not live within a reasonable proximity to the coast.

Clearly, some elements of the surfing experience will be lost in a tightly controlled environment like a surf park, however, they offer greatly enhanced levels of safety, guaranteed optimal surfing conditions, easy access into the pool, poolside amenities, and exponentially more wave riding time thereby facilitating increased participant access to surf therapy.

References

Anderson, J. (2013). Cathedrals of the surf zone: Regulating access to a space of spirituality. *Social & Cultural Geography, 14*(8), 954–972.

Armitano, C., Clapham, E. D., Audette, J., & Lamont, L. (2015). Benefits of surfing for children with disabilities: A pilot study. *Palaestra, 29*, 31–34.

A Walk on Water [AWOW]. (n.d.). What happens at an AWOW event? Retrieved June 10, 2019 from https://awalkonwater.org/faq/

A Walk on Water [AWOW]. (2018). Autism utopia. Retrieved June 9, 2019 from https://awalkonwater.org/autism-utopia/

Best Day Foundation. (n.d.[a]). Surf Chair 200. Retrieved from June 10, 2019 https://bestdayfoundation.org/surfchair-2000/

Best Day Foundation (n.d.[b]). Check out what our fans are saying. Retrieved June 10, 2019 from https://bestdayfoundation.org/

Butts, S. (2001). Good to the last drop: Understanding surfers' motivations [Electronic Version]. *Sociology of Sport Online, 4*. Retrieved July 18, 2019 from http://physed.otago.ac.nz/sosol

Caddick, N., Phoenix, C., & Smith, B. (2015a). Collective stories and well-being: Using a dialogical narrative approach to understand peer relationships among combat veterans experiencing post-traumatic stress disorder. *Journal of Health Psychology, 20*(3), 286–299.

Caddick, N., Smith, B., & Phoenix, C. (2015b). The effects of surfing and the natural environment on the well-being of combat veterans. *Qualitative Health Research, 25*(1), 76–86.

Cavanaugh, L. K. & Rademacher, S. B. (2014). How a surfing social skills curriculum can impact children with autism spectrum disorders. *Journal of the International Association of Special Education, 15*(1), 27–35.

Clapham, E. D., Armitano, C. N., Lamont, L. S., & Audette, J. G. (2014). The ocean as a unique therapeutic environment: Developing a surfing program. *Journal of Physical Education, Recreation and Dance, 85*(4), 8–14.

Colpus, S. & Taylor, J. (2014). Ride every challenge: The impact of surfing on 100 young people facing personal and emotional challenges. *British Journal of Sports Medicine, 48*, 1581–1582.

Coon, J. T., Boddy, K., Stein, K., Whear, R., Barton, J., & Depledge, M. (2011). Does participating in physical activity in outdoor natural environments have a greater effect on physical and mental wellbeing than physical activity indoors? A systematic review. *Environmental Science and Technology, 17*, 379–388.

Crawford, P. & Wright, R. (1994). The quest to find the first surfer in the world. *Australian Surfer, 1*, 4–6.

Crawford, R. (2016). *The impact of ocean therapy on veterans with posttraumatic stress disorder* (Unpublished doctoral dissertation). Grand Canyon University, Phoenix, AZ.

Dawson, K. (2018). *Undercurrents of power: Aquatic culture in the African diaspora*. Philadelphia, PA: University of Pennsylvania Press.

Depledge, M. & Bird, W. (2009). The blue gym: Health and wellbeing from our coasts. *Marine Pollution Bulletin, 58*, 947–948.

Devine-Wright, H. & Godfrey, C. (2018). *Surf therapy: The long-term impact*. Newquay, England: The Wave Project.

Dustin, D. L., Bricker, K., Negley, S., Brownlee, M., Schwab, K. A., & Lundberg, N. (Eds.) (2016). *This land is your land: Toward a better understanding of nature's resiliency-building and restorative power for armed forces*. Urbana, IL: Sagamore Venture Publishing.

Farmer, R. J. (1992). Surfing: Motivations, values, and culture. *Journal of Sport Behavior, 15*(3), 231–257.

Fleischmann, D., Michalewicz, B., Stedje-Larsen, E., Neff, J., Murphy, J., Browning, K., ..., & Mclay, R. (2011). Surf medicine: Surfing as a means of therapy for combat-related polygram. *Journal of Prosthetics and Orthotics, 23*(1), 2–29.

Gaspar de Matos, M., Santos, A., Fauvelet, C., Marta, F., Evangelista, E. S., Ferreira, J., & Moita, M. (2017). Surfing for social integration: Mental health and well-being promotion through surf therapy among institutionalized young people. *HSOA Journal of Community Medicine and Public Health Care, 4*(1), 1–6.

Giddens, A. (1991). *Modernity and self-identity*. Cambridge, MA: Polity.

Godfrey, C., Devine-Wright, H., & Taylor, J. (2015). The positive impact of structured surfing courses on the wellbeing of vulnerable young people. *Community Practitioner, 88*(1), 26–29.

Harris, K. B. (2015) *Working with addiction through surf therapy: A phenomenological exploration of healing* (Unpublished Master's thesis). Pacifica Graduate Institute, Santa Barbara, CA.

Hignett, A., White, M. P., Pahl, S., Jenkin, R., & Le Froy, M. (2017). Evaluation of a surfing programme designed to increase personal well-being and connectedness to the natural environment among 'at risk' young people, *Journal of Adventure Education and Outdoor Learning, 18*(1), 53–69.

International Surfing Association [ISA]. (2017). ISA adaptive surfing sport classes. Retrieved June 10, 2019 from http://www.isasurf.org/wp-content/uploads/downloads/2017/06/2017-ISA-Adaptive-Surfing-Classification-Updated.pdf

International Surf Therapy Organization [ISTO]. (2019). International surf therapy organization: Go far together. Retrieved August 1, 2019 from https://intlsurftherapy.org/

Jones, W. (2017, July 12). Maine's special surfers organization goes all in with 'immersion'. *Eastern Surf Magazine*. Retrieved June 10, 2019 from https://www.easternsurf.com/news/special-surfers-immersion/

Lambert, C. (2019) *Waves of healing: How surfing changes the lives of children with autism*. Hobart, NY: Hatherleigh Press.

Lanagan, D. (2002). Surfing in the third millennium: Commodifying the visual argot. *The Australian Journal of Anthropology, 13*(3), 283–291.

Michalewicz-Kragh, B. (2019) *Evaluation of outcomes following surf therapy*. Retrieved June 10, 2019 from https://clinicaltrials.gov/ct2/show/NCT028 57751

Moore, A. M., Clapham, E. D., & Deeney, T. A. (2018). Parents' perspectives on surf therapy for children with disabilities. *International Journal of Disability, Development and Education, 65*(3), 304–317.

Nerothin, P. H. (2018). *A phenomenological investigation of lifestyle surfers from San Diego* (Unpublished master's thesis). Prescott College, Prescott, AZ.

Nichols, W. J. (2014). *Blue mind: The surprising science that shows how being near, in, on, or under water can make you happier, healthier, more connected, and better at what you do*. New York, NY: Little Brown Spark.

O'Brien, D. & Eddie, I. (2013). *Benchmarking global best practice: Innovation and leadership in surf city tourism and industry development*. Paper presented at the Global Surf Cities Conference, Gold Coast, Australia.

O'Brien, D. & Ponting, J. (2013). Sustainable surf tourism: A community centered approach in Papua New Guinea. *Journal of Sport Management, 27*, 158–172.

Pearson, K. (1979). *Surfing subcultures of Australia and New Zealand*. St Lucia, Australia: University of Queensland Press.

Ponting, J. & O'Brien, D. (2013). Liberalizing Nirvana: An analysis of the consequences of common pool resource deregulation for the sustainability of Fiji's surf tourism industry. *Journal of Sustainable Tourism, 22*(3), 384–402.

Ponting, J. (2017). Simulating Nirvana: Surf parks, surfing spaces, and sustainability. In G. Borne & J. Ponting (Eds.), *Sustainable surfing* (pp. 219–237). New York, NY: Routledge.

Ride a Wave. (n.d.). About us. Retrieved from http://www.rideawave.org/about_ride_a_wave.php

Roberts, M. & Ponting, J. (2018). Waves of simulation: Arguing authenticity in an era of surfing the hyperreal. *International Review for the Sociology of Sport*, 55(2), 1–17.

Rogers, C. M., Mallinson, T., & Peppers, D. (2014). High-intensity sports for posttraumatic stress disorder and depression: Feasibility study of ocean therapy with veterans of Operation Enduring Freedom and Operation Iraqi Freedom. *The American Journal of Occupational Therapy*, 68(4), 395–404.

Stranger, M. (1999). The aesthetics of risk: A study of surfing. *International Review for the Sociology of Sport*, 34(3), 256–276.

Stranger, M. (2011). *Surfing life: Surface, substructure and the commodification of the sublime*. Farnham, England: Ashgate.

Stuhl, A. & Porter, H. (2015). Riding the waves: Therapeutic surfing to improve social skills for children with autism. *Therapeutic Recreation Journal*, 49(3), 253–254.

Surfers Healing. (n.d.). History. Retrieved 2 August, 2019 from https://www.surfershealing.org/history

Taylor, B. (2007). Surfing into spirituality and a new, aquatic nature religion. *Journal of the American Academy of Religion*, 75(4), 923–951.

Walker, I. H. (2011). *Waves of resistance: Surfing and history in 20th century Hawai'i*. Honolulu, HI: University of Hawaii Press.

Warshaw, M. (2004). *The encyclopedia of surfing*. New York, NY: Penguin Books.

White, M. Smith, A., Humphreys, K., Pahl, S., Snelling, D. & Depledge, M. (2010). Blue Space: The importance of water for preference, effect, and restorativeness rating of natural and built scenes. *Journal of Environmental Psychology*, 30, 482–493.

World Surf League [WSL]. (n.d.). Sponsorship: The World Surf League - A partnership like no other. Retrieved June 10, 2019 from http://www.worldsurfleague.com/pages/sponsorship

Chapter 13

Forest Therapy

Won Sop Shin and Juyoung Lee

Shin to bul ee ~ Body and soil are one.

Ancient Korean Proverb

Introduction and Background

The therapeutic effects of time spent in a forest can be considered an environmental health treatment. Research reviews and formally developed clinical practices now support the reality that forests provide opportunities to foster more efficient and active behavior in patients, thereby enhancing mental and physical health and psychological functioning (Hansen, Jones, & Tocchini, 2017; Shin, Yeoun, Yoo, & Shin, 2010). This approach, more than any other expressed in this book, is currently receiving significant attention in mainstream literature and health practices as evidenced by a simple review of new books. Using the search terms forest therapy, forest bathing, or *shinrin yoku* (Japanese term for forest bathing), you will find more than 15 new manuscripts published in 2018 and 2019 alone. They range from simple, non-clinical expressions of mindful practices in nature, through to well-researched and authoritative descriptions (e.g., Li, 2019). This chapter is based on the research and practice of forest therapy (known in Korea as *sanlimyok*). Forest therapy has been developed and studied intensively in Korea from the perspective of the authors, experienced and leading researchers on the topic of forest therapy and as a former minister of the Korean Forest Service (first author).

Those living in urban areas may have experienced increased disconnect from natural environments due to rapid development of human constructed spaces and hurried lifestyles. This has been posited to have an adverse effect on humankind (Nisbet & Zelenski, 2011). When seen from the viewpoint of urban environmental change, environmental problems such as atmospheric and water pollution are now a factor that directly threatens our lives. We are also exposed to diverse environmental stresses in urban settings, such as noise pollution and excessive lighting that prevent a clear vision of the night sky. In fact, we may not recognize these impacts when born into them and conditioned by city living (Falchi, Cinzano, Elvidge, Keith, & Haim, 2011).

Natural environments were the basis of life and places of production for human beings in the past, as well as central features in religious and shamanistic practice (Clifford, 2018). Considering the length of human existence, the rapidly experienced changes in our technological, economic, and social structures related to natural environments may be some of the causes of our ill health (Gluckman, Hanson, & Spencer, 2005). Forest therapy is premised on reconnecting humans to the natural environment through stimulation of our senses (e.g., aromatics from soil and essential oils from trees, etc.) and the resulting health benefits.

Forests can play unique roles as restorative and healing places able to clear our minds and provide psychological stability and mental healing effects (Shin et al., 2010). These places now enable urbanites who are hungry for reconnection to feel the preciousness of nature. That is, thanks to considerable efforts by a group of dedicated Korean researchers and government officials, forests are now places where the essence of nature is relatively well preserved and can be relatively easily accessed by those whose lives are isolated from nature due to industrialization and urbanization (Korea Forest Welfare Institute, 2018).

Target Populations

Forest therapy can be ideal for those who want improve their health, those who want mental and physical recovery, rest, or to simply improve their quality of life. Park (2015) considered it a broad general health intervention through the treatment of diagnosed psychological to many medical issues. Although healthy people may commonly use forests for recreation, those who use these environments to maintain and manage their health would be included as the population ideal for forest therapy.

For those who want to improve and maintain health, and are not experiencing the occurrence of disease, they are still recommended to partake in forest therapy activities that promote health rather than relying on medicine or the formal health care system (Korea Forest Welfare Institute, 2018). Therefore, the purpose of forest therapy programs in general can be said to promote mental and physical health, or to improve human health by utilizing forest environments (Park, 2015).

Patients with cardiovascular disease, diabetes, depression, or mild cognitive impairments have included forest therapy as part of their medical care (Li, 2019; Park, 2015). As with health supplement foods taken by patients as a means of assistance to improve treatment effects while taking medicines prescribed by medical workers, voluntarily participating in forest therapy programs provide assistance to improve the effects of treatments being received at medical institutions.

Key Developments

Traditionally, timber has been the material obtained from forests representing the economic value of forests. Humans have historically used timber for fuel, building materials, firewood, tool making, and the fabrication of means of transportation. In the traditional era, forests were a sort of raw material warehouses.

Much of Korea is now an urban society and to combat the disconnection from nature, many have sought out the forest setting and to partake in forest activities which provide both preventive and therapeutic health benefits (Kaplan, 1995). Extensive research has provided empirical evidence that a forest experience, or even the viewing of forest scenes, contributes to reducing stress, promoting more positive moods and feelings, and may facilitate recovery from illness (Shin, 1993, 2007; Shin & Kim, 2007; Shin & Oh, 1996).

To institutionalize healing forests, the Korean Forestry Culture and Recreation Act was amended in 2010. Through the amendment, the definition of 'healing forest' was newly established, grounds for the standards, procedures, and the development of healing forests and facilities were prepared. In addition, to prepare for effective utilization of forest therapy, the concept of forest therapy, the forest therapy instructor system, and the designation of training institutes for forest therapy instructors were revised.

In 2014, the Korean Forestry Culture and Recreation Act was amended to expand the scope of activities of forest therapy instructors, which was limited to the existing healing forests, to include natural recreational forests, forest bathing parks, and forest paths. The Act was amended to enable experts in forest education, such as forest interpreters and early childhood forest instructors to acquire the license of a forest therapy instructor after attaining three years' experience post-licensure. In addition, the regulation for the healing forest area standard for minimum size for metropolitan areas was relaxed from at least 300,000 m^2 to at least 150,000 m^2, so that the development of healing forests in cities could be increased to enable the expansion of forest therapy services.

To systematically describe the direction of development of forest therapy, the Korea Forest Service set its vision as "national health promotion through the activation of forest therapy" in 2012 through the collection of diverse opinions of experts and consultants, and established the "forest therapy activation promotion plan" consisting of specific tasks for "the construction and expansion of forest therapy infrastructures" (Korea Forest Welfare Institute, 2016).

Discussion of Practice

Modern urban life can produce a high-tension state in humans and people may easily accept the notion of spending time in forest environments to recover our senses. The relief felt in a forest can enhance our level of immunity, making our bodies increasingly resistant to diseases, and more readily to recover from diseases (Hartig, Mitchell, De Vries, & Frumkin, 2014). The environmental elements of forests, which can be represented by the scenery, smell, and sound of forests, can stimulate the five senses of humans so that humans can easily sympathize with natural environments in forests. In addition to the five-sensory stimuli, factors such as phytoncide, anion elements, and photo-environmental elements are also elements of forest therapy (Li, 2019).

The color green, and forest scenery can relieve the fatigue of the eyes and bring about the stability of mind (Akers et al., 2012). In addition, the diverse natural colors and landscapes are known to have the effect to inhibit the secretion of the stress hormone cortisol by soothing the fatigue of an exhausted mind and body. This can invite emotional and physical stability by suppressing the sympathetic nervous system and activating the parasympathetic nervous system in the autonomic nervous system. Therefore, the brain is stabilized and *alpha*-waves, which are generated when comfortable, can be significantly increased in forest environments (Lee, Shin, Yeoun, & Yoo, 2009).

Phytoncide is the compound of 'phyton' meaning plants, and 'cide' meaning killer. Phytoncide is known to help regulate immunity, and is antibacterial, anti-inflammatory, insecticidal, antiviral, spasmolytic, anti-hyperglycemic, anticancer, antiallergic, and has sterilizing effects (Li et al., 2009). Phytoncide is utilized in diverse fields, such as pharmaceutical products, hygiene products, cosmetics, and the food industry in the field of microorganisms. Recently, phytoncide has been found to relax tension when inhaled in the form of a fragrance and reduce the concentration of stress hormones in the body when taken as a food additive (Li et al., 2009).

Anion elements are massively generated in the process of photosynthesis to inhale carbon dioxide and produce oxygen in forests and are also abundant in waterfalls and valleys in general. Anions are produced during photosynthesis, making them abundant in forests. In fact, there is evidence to suggest that the number of anions present in forests is 800–2,000 parts per cubic centimeter, which is 14–70 times the number of anions present indoors in cities (Wu, Wang, Xu, & Hu, 2007). When there are more than 1,000 anions parts per cubic centimeter, *alpha*-waves act vigorously to relieve tension, and anion-rich air may relieve headaches and inhibit free histamine, a neurohormone found to cause respiratory diseases.

Sunlight activates the secretion of serotonin that makes us happy and enables vitamin D synthesis in our body (Lambert, Reid, Kaye, Jennings, &

Esler, 2002). When the amount of sunlight is reduced, we can be less energetic, and our mind and body may become lethargic, leading to subdued moods. Sunlight in forests does not beat down on our body, but mostly indirectly reaches our body after being reflected by forest components like the leaves possibly reducing exposure to ultraviolet rays.

Oxygen is an essential element for all living things, including human beings and forests are huge oxygen factories. In general, the concentration of oxygen in the air is about 21% in cities and about 2% less in indoor and about 2% higher in forests (Schreml et al., 2010). The clean oxygen present in forests is said to have excellent effects in preventing and treating various diseases such as cancer, maintaining youthful skin, and brain activation. The sounds produced in forests, such as the music of birds or the sounds of water and wind, are natural rhythms that can stabilize our body and mind, correcting lost biorhythms and restoring health and vitality (Thoma et al., 2013).

Forest therapy programs can be applied and divided to a range of visitors coming to healing forests, such as patients with specific diseases or healthy citizens among the general public. Programs are premised on the use of forest therapy resources and forest environmental elements, and are purposed to promote mental and physical health. After analyzing a total of 521 forest therapy programs, the programs were identified as fitting into a number of categories such as walking, exercise, meditation, art, play, cooking, education, counseling/psychotherapy, and planting (Forest Therapy Research Project Group, 2018).

Theory, Research, and Efficacy

Attention Restoration Theory proposes that exposure to nature, such as a forest, reduces mental fatigue or, more precisely, directed attention fatigue. A theory attempting to explain these effects, proposed by Kaplan (1995) suggests prolonged use of directed attention leads to the fatigue of neural mechanisms. The recovery of effective functioning is enabled by settings that have certain key components, such as being away, extent, fascination, and compatibility; key properties of forests that trigger mental processes or states contributing to restorative experiences (Laumann, Gärling, & Stormark, 2001).

Psycho Evolutionary Theory explains how natural environments relieve stress responses (Ulrich, 1983; Ulrich et al., 1991). Unlike attention restoration theory, this theory deals with the positive effects of natural environments on human beings from the viewpoint of evolution of mankind. Humans have evolved in natural environments for a long period of time and are therefore adapted to show psychologically and physiologically more positive responses to natural environments than to urban environments (Gluckman et al., 2005). Natural environments provided food and shelter for humans to survive resulting in positive feelings toward nature. In other words, preferring and responding positively to natural environments was advantageous for human survival and prosperity, hence the genetic tendency to pay attention to natural environments appeared (Ulrich et al., 1991).

Ulrich et al. (1991) also developed a Stress Recovery Theory from the evolutionary psychological point of view related to natural environments. Stress recovery theory argued that natural environments are important for the maintenance of positive functions of humans, and discusses how natural elements can play important roles in recovery from stress. Ulrich (1993) further stated that when under stress, the human body naturally begins physiological responses in order to create positive emotions by regulating physiological effects and recharging the energy to cope with stress responses. From the evolutionary psychological viewpoint, this theory indicates that nature provides the elements necessary for the survival of human beings and helps humans adapt to natural environments. That is, positive responses to nature occur when nature provides the primordial functions needed for humans' survival.

Outcome Studies

From the beginning of the mid-2000s, studies on the health benefits directly provided by forests to humans have been conducted in earnest although studies on the effects of diverse environmental elements have been conducted since 1980. Through efforts, such as measuring the physiological and psychological responses of the human body to diverse forest environments, the health benefits of forest therapy have become objectively verifiable and moving research findings into the realm of evidence-based medicine (Hansen et al., 2017; Park et al., 2010). As the effects of forest environments on human mind and body became to be measured in objective and verifiable methods, forest therapy has gained social trust in Korea (and elsewhere) and continues to build its reputation upon this research.

Studies on forest therapy are building a new discipline that blends forests and human well-being in diverse fields such as sociology, psychology, and health science as well as forestry. As for studies in the field of forest therapy, they have been conducted across these diverse fields and are beginning to shape a clear picture of the psychological, physiological, and physical effects of forests and natural environments on human beings.

Studies of Psychological and Mental Effects of Forest Therapy

Studies on the effects of programs using the healing functions of forests were mainly conducted in the fields of psychology and psychiatry.

Although forest therapy programs vary in their target populations and practices, most studies report the effects of forest therapy programs positively indicating that forest therapy programs practically have significant potential in the areas personal growth including self-concept and the promotion of positive human relations.

Miyazaki, Motohashi, and Kobayashi (1992) showed that negative emotions such as depression, anxiety, and hostility are reduced, and positive emotions increase in forest environments compared to artificial air-conditioned rooms. Song, Shin, Yeoun and Choi (2009) indicated that in a forest therapy program for single mothers, depression decreased drastically, and self-esteem improved significantly. Lee and Jeong (2011) had patients with chronic schizophrenia participate in a forest experience program for eight weeks to check the healing effects and identified positive effects in the form of significant improvement of all of depressive symptoms, positive coping with negative thoughts, and description of emotions. You, Kim, Lee, Jang, and Son (2014) identified that a mental health program utilizing forest bathing had effects to positively improve the depression resolution of adult women and to improve psychological well-being. In addition, Shin et al. (2015) indicated that job stress decreased, the mood state elements such as tension-anxiety, depression, anger, difficulties, and fatigue decreased significantly, and vigor increased significantly. Park et al. (2017) could identify that teachers' stress response index and the sub areas such as physical symptoms, depressive symptoms, and anger symptoms were lowered with the mental health program utilizing forest bathing and the program was effective in relieving negative feelings. Lee, Yeoun, Park, and Gang (2018) reported that the program was effective in relieving stress, improving positive emotions, and resolving negative feelings of emotional workers.

Studies of Physiological Effects of Forest Therapy

Physiological changes are indicators of important health-related effects of forest use. More generally speaking, the effects of physiological changes are a variable directly associated with physical or mental well-being, and changes in heart rate, blood pressure, and brain waves are considered to be variables that can directly predicate the psychological or physical health of humans.

In a scientific empirical survey on the health and healing effects of forests, healthy adult male subjects spent a number of days in an urban environment and a forest environment, respectively, and blood and urine tests were carried out thereafter (Li et al., 2008). The results indicated the NK cells (white blood cells which have cancer-fighting and immune function properties) were activated and levels of adrenaline present in the urine (stress indicator) were reduced, both significantly. Further, these effects were maintained for seven days following the forest experience while the urban control showed neither of these benefits.

A South Korean study (Park et al., 2010) conducted to investigate the physiological effects of forest bathing, asked the subjects to appreciate forest and urban landscapes for 15 minutes and measured the heart rate variability and blood pressure of the subjects as physiological indicators. The researchers could obtain a finding that the subjects' systolic blood pressure and heart rate variability of the subjects were significantly lower when they were appreciating forest landscapes compared to when they were appreciating urban landscapes. In addition, heart rate variability was significantly higher when they were appreciating forest landscapes. In order to clarify the effect of the visual environment of the forest on the psychology and physiology of the human body, Lee et al. (2009) presented visual environments in which a city, a forest, or forest and water exist and measured physiological and psychological changes using *alpha*-waves, the Perceived Restorativeness Scale, and the Positive and Negative Affect Schedule scale. As a result, natural environments were found to be more positively evaluated than urban environments, and that among the visual environments of nature, rather than those visual environments where only forests were present, those visual environments where forests and water coexist were more positively evaluated. Kim and Park (2016) reported that after a forest therapy exercise program, *alpha*-waves and *beta*-waves increased to improve brain health.

Studies of Physical Health Effects of Forest Therapy

Among studies that investigated the exercise effects of forest therapy, Choi et al. (2016) indicated that forest exercise was more effective in increasing HDL-cholesterol and reducing triglyceride than in indoor exercise and affected increases in SOD and melatonin concentrations. According to Lee and Shin (2015), forest walking meditation decreased middle-aged women's tension, depression, and confusion, and affective self-awareness increased while feelings of being judged decreased. Choi, Shin, and Yeoun (2014) also identified that after forest walking exercise, elderly persons showed more significant improvement in leg strength, waist flexibility, agility/dynamic balance, cardiopulmonary endurance, walking rhythm, walking speed, and gait stability. Further, in a forest exercise study conducted by Lee, Yeoun, and Choi (2016), elderly females showed significant improvement in knee joint muscle strength, muscle endurance, and bone density of the lumbar spine and the intertrochanteric region. Kwon and Choi (2016) derived implications for the realization of the forest elderly welfare service through case studies and analysis of previous studies.

Case Vignette: National Forest Healing Complex

In South Korea, efforts to recover health and improve the quality of life have increased since 2005 due to changes in living environments resulting from the improvement of income levels and rapid urbanization, increases in the burden of medical expenses, increases in environmental disease, and increases in environment stress. Among them, forest therapy has begun to receive attention. Plans to utilize forest therapy have been sought, and related efforts began with the implementation of a planned project from the Korea Forest Service in 2007, which was supervised by the Korea Forest Research Institute. As of 2018, there are 51 healing forests nationwide (22 in operation at time of writing and 29 being constructed) with more than a million visitors with approximately 8.7% of all visitors participating in diverse healing forests programs. The Korea Forest Welfare Institute, a public organization responsible for the practical work of the forest welfare services has established Health Promotion Centers in the forests to increase program activity and participation levels of forest therapy.

The National Forest Healing Complex (hereafter, the complex) is a hub facility for forest healing involved in research and development, education, and long-term stay in forest healing facilities, which was made to improve human health and increase quality of life by using an abundance of forest resources. The complex is located in the northeast of Korea and has 2,889 ha of total area in a protected mountain area. More than ~US$130 million was invested in this six-year project from the national budget and completed in 2015. The site has varied altitudes ranging from 400 to 1,000 m and has a variety of mountain terrain, microclimates, and vegetation compositions, which provide diverse forest healing experiences. This area has been conserved for a long time and the forest is well developed, with diverse ecosystem of plant and animal species.

The area of the complex is divided largely into two zones, the central zone and the forest zone. There are many different facilities in the core zone, including the health promotion center, visitor center, hydrotherapy center, meditation center, auditorium, several types of healing gardens, lodges for short- and long-term stays, restaurants, a small library, several walking paths, and small waterfronts. The forest zone is comprised of multiple places for meditation, physical exercise, viewing scenery, and different types of trails totaling 60 km in length designed for walking, sports activities, mountain climbing, and historic and cultural experiences. A universal design was applied to each facility for easy access. A 2 km, gently-sloping path made of timber is available for use by people in wheelchairs, parents with baby strollers, and those with physical disabilities.

When planning this project, the target groups were mainly people with chronic, environmental, and lifestyle-related diseases, such as hypertension, diabetes, depression, atopic dermatitis, ADHD, and so on. Additionally, a more general group of people in need of stress release or a healthy lifestyle was also identified as a target market for the complex. Evidence-based healing programs provided by certified forest healing instructors were developed to provide high quality experiences for many different groups of people. Exercise specialists prescribe physical exercise programs for individuals who need customized healing programs that includes indoor and outdoor training. Aquatic healing programs are also provided in a hydrotherapy center that includes a pool, spa, and sauna facilities for individuals in need of physical therapy, injury rehabilitation, therapeutic exercise, or functional training. For all users, a healthy diet is provided to reduce caloric intake and promote weight loss. The complex is also expected to play a key role in providing continuing professional education for forest healing instructors in collaboration with academic and practical specialists in the fields of medicine, psychology, counselling, management, tourism, and marketing.

The five-sense experience in the forest is a program to recover dulled senses through the stimulation of the forest with a walk to experience relaxation of the body and mind. The five sense experiences include visual, auditory, olfactory, taste and touch. In the visual experience, the participants are encouraged to naturally walk through the forest, while looking at the nearest and farthest places, finding what attracts them particularly, and have time to think about why they were attracted by it. In the auditory sense experience, the participants hear diverse sounds of forests, such as birdsongs, the sound of water, or the sound of winds, and shares opinions regarding differences between everyday sounds and the sounds of forests. The olfactory sense experience is an activity to firsthand relate to the fragrance of the forest.

Meditation in the forest can help participants to reach a state of calm, to relieve stress, and to reflect on themselves. Participants are invited to concentrate on inhalation and exhalation while engaging their senses in the forest. Barefoot walking is another example of a forest activity. This activity can help one recover one's senses and alleviate stress in order to relax the body and mind. The participants are invited to select a forest trail, remove their shoes, and walk slowly barefoot along the trail. Barefoot walking is known to be effective for maintaining balance of the body, strengthening muscles, improving blood circulation, posture correction, relieving low back pain, and reducing blood pressure. However, there are precautions; barefoot walking should be conducted slowly because it takes time to become familiar with the practice and those who have mobility issues or other contraindications should be screened in advance and only participate as they can.

Discussion

Globally, forest policies are facing a paradigm shift. As diverse environmental issues have emerged, the viewpoint should be changed to look differently at forests in terms of human sustainability. In the constant changes of industrialization and urbanization, rapid transition to a technological and information society is taking place. This leads to changes in the way we see the environment and suggests a new perspective is needed on policy choices for the forest sector moving forward.

Based on the experiences and development of forest therapy in Korea, we propose the forest should be evaluated as a welfare resource beyond the existing framework for forest products and environment preservation. First, the relationships between forests and humans is reestablished. Preserving forests can lead to human welfare and create a virtuous cycle structure in which forests are better preserved and cultivated to obtain better quality welfare benefits. Compared to social welfare in which services are provided through redistribution of consumable goods, the case of forest welfare, services are obtained through well-cultivated nature. Therefore, it imposes little burden on national finances, and anyone can enjoy the benefits of these services regardless of social class, age, or gender to improve the quality of life and happiness of individuals.

Hippocrates, who is often referred to as the founder of modern medicine, said "It is the basis of medicine to nurture the natural healing power or immunity of the human body." The health function of the forest raises our immunity, thereby enabling us not only to prevent diseases but also to assist in curing disease. Cities, home to many in the world, are filled with numerous health threatening factors (i.e., pollution, noise, artificial light, etc.) which dull our senses and expose us to diseases. In addition, the serious stress that modern people experience can cause various mental/physical diseases. Forests can rescue us from environmental pollution and revitalize our senses that have become dull in urban life so that our health is restored. In addition, an important function for health of the forest is the role of buffering and mitigating the stress that we experience.

Forests are an indispensable resource capable of revealing our identity enabling us to have the essence and meaning of life beyond the economic resources they provide us with. Those who live in modern urban spaces are almost completely disconnected from the forest which our body and mind crave. That is why we need forests. By accessing forests frequently, we can live as human beings should, in relationship with nature. Our instincts and potential abilities can be enlivened through the forest and thereby we can live as healthier, happier, and self-realized lives.

References

Akers, A., Barton, J., Cossey, R., Gainsford, P., Griffin, M., & Micklewright, D. (2012). Visual color perception in green exercise: Positive effects on mood and perceived exertion. *Environmental Science & Technology, 46*(16), 8661–8666.

Choi, J. H., Ryu, K. H., Kim, T. S., Shin, C. S., Yeoun, P. S., & Kim, H. J. (2016). Effects of 12-week forest exercise on blood lipids, SOD, and melatonin in the middle-aged women. *The Journal of Korean Institute of Forest Recreation, 20*(4), 81–90.

Choi, J. H., Shin, C. S., & Yeoun, P. S. (2014). Effects of forest-walking exercise on functional fitness and gait pattern in the elderly. *Journal of Korean Forest Society, 103*(3), 503–509.

Clifford, M. A. (2018). *Your guide to forest bathing: Experience the healing power of nature.* Newburyport, MA: Conari Press.

Falchi, F., Cinzano, P., Elvidge, C. D., Keith, D. M., & Haim, A. (2011). Limiting the impact of light pollution on human health, environment and stellar visibility. *Journal of Environmental Management, 92*(10), 2714–2722.

Forest Therapy Research Project Group. (2018). *Understanding of forest therapy.* Seoul, Korea.

Gluckman, P. D., Hanson, M. A., & Spencer, H. G. (2005). Predictive adaptive responses and human evolution. *Trends in Ecology & Evolution, 20*(10), 527–533.

Hansen, M. M., Jones, R., & Tocchini, K. (2017). Shinrin-yoku (forest bathing) and nature therapy: A state-of-the-art review. *International Journal of Environmental Research and Public Health, 14*(8), 851.

Hartig, T., Mitchell, R., De Vries, S., & Frumkin, H. (2014). Nature and health. *Annual Review of Public Health, 35*, 207–228.

Kaplan, S. (1995). The restorative benefits of nature: Toward an integrative framework. *Journal of Environmental Psychology, 15*, 169–82.

Kim, B. G. & Park, I. S. (2016). The effects of forest therapy on brain waves. *Korea Entertainment Industry Association*, 211–214.

Korea Forest Welfare Institute. (2016). *The last decade of forest therapy.* Daejeon, Korea.

Korea Forest Welfare Institute. (2018). *Introduction of forest-welfare.* Daejeon, Korea.

Kwon, G, C. & Choi, J. S. (2016). Forest healing program development for realization of forest welfare service for the elderly on the aging society. *Journal of The Korean Society of Beauty and Arts, 17*(1), 249–263.

Lambert, G. W., Reid, C., Kaye, D. M., Jennings, G. L., & Esler, M. D. (2002). Effect of sunlight and season on serotonin turnover in the brain. *The Lancet, 360*(9348), 1840–1842.

Laumann, K., Gärling, T., & Stormark, K. M. (2001). Rating scale measures of restorative components of environment. *Journal of Environmental Psychology, 21*(1), 31–44.

Lee, G. M. & Jeong, Y. C. (2011). Effects of the forest healing program on schizophrenia. *Korean Forest Society*, 467–469.

Lee, J. H., Shin, W. S., Yeoun, P. S., & Yoo, R. H. (2009). The influence of forest scenes on psychophysiolosical responses. *Journal of Korean Forestry Society, 98*(1), 88–93.

Lee, J. S., Yeoun, P. S., & Choi, J. H. (2016). Effects of forest walking exercise on isokinetic muscular strength, muscular endurance, and bone mineral density in the elderly women. *The Journal of Korean Institute of Forest Recreation, 20*(1), 1–9.

Lee, J. W., Yeoun, P. S., Park, S. H., & Gang, J. W. (2018). Effects of forest therapy programs on the stress and emotional change of emotional labor workers. *The Journal of Korean Institute of Forest Recreation, 22*(3), 15–22.

Lee, Y, J. & Shin, C. S. (2015). Effects of forest walking meditation on mood states and self-awareness in middle-aged women. *The Journal of Korean Institute of Forest Recreation, 19*(3), 19–25.

Li, Q. (2019). *Forest bathing: How trees can help you find health and happiness.* New York, NY: Viking.

Li, Q., Morimoto, K., Kobayashi, M., Inagaki, H., Katsumata, M., Hirata, Y., ... & Kawada, T. (2008). Visiting a forest, but not a city, increases human natural killer activity and expression of anti-cancer proteins. *International Journal of Immunopathology and Pharmacology, 21*(1), 117–127.

Li, Q., Kobayashi, M., Wakayama, Y., Inagaki, H., Katsumata, M., Hirata, Y., ..., & Ohira, T. (2009). Effect of phytoncide from trees on human natural killer cell function. *International Journal of Immunopathology and Pharmacology, 22*(4), 951–959.

Miyazaki, Y., Motohashi, Y., & Kobayashi, S. (1992). A change of mood caused by the inhalation of oil refining. Effects of daylighting, workability, sensory tests and psychological condition evaluation. *Wood Research Society, 38*(10), 903–908.

Nisbet, E. K. & Zelenski, J. M. (2011). Underestimating nearby nature: Affective forecasting errors obscure the happy path to sustainability. *Psychological Science, 22*(9), 1101–1106.

Park, B. J. (2015). *Understanding natural resources (Forest therapy).* Seoul, Korea.

Park, B. J., Kasetani, T., Morikawa, T., Tsunetsugu, Y., Kagawa, T., & Miyazaki, Y. (2010). The physiological effects of Shinrin-yoku (taking in the forest atmosphere or forest bathing): Evidence from field experiments in 24 forests across Japan. *Environmental Health and Preventative Medicine, 15*(1), 18–26.

Park, S. H., Yeon, P. S., Hong, C. W., Yeo, E. H., Han, S. M., Lee, H. Y., ..., Kim, Y. H. (2017). A study on the effect of the forest healing programs on teachers' stress and PANAS. *Korean Journal of Environment and Ecology, 31*(6), 606–614.

Schreml, S., Szeimies, R. M., Prantl, L., Karrer, S., Landthaler, M., & Babilas, P. (2010). Oxygen in acute and chronic wound healing. *British Journal of Dermatology, 163*(2), 257–268.

Shin, C. S., Yeoun, P. S., Kim, Y. G., Eum, J. O., Yim, Y. R., Yoon, S. B., ..., Lee, S. H. (2015). The influence of a forest healing program on public servants in charge of social welfare and mental health care worker's job stress and the profile of mood states. *Journal of the Korean Forestry Society, 104*(2), 294–299.

Shin, W. S. (1993). The understanding of forest campers' attitudes and their self-actualization (in Korean). *Journal of Korean Forest Society, 82,* 107–121.

Shin, W. S. (2007). The influence of forest view through a window on job satisfaction and job stress. *Scandanavian Journal of Forest Research, 22,* 248–253.

Shin, W. S. & Kim, S. K. (2007). The influence of forest experience on alcoholics' depression levels (in Korean). *Journal of Korean Forest Society, 96,* 203–207.

Shin, W. S. & Oh, H. K. (1996). The influence of forest program on depression levels (in Korean). *Journal of Korean Forest Society, 85,* 586–595.

Shin, W. S., Yeoun, P. S., Yoo, R. W., & Shin, C. S. (2010). Forest experience and psychological health benefits: The state of the art and future prospect in Korea. *Environmental Health and Preventive Medicine, 15*(1), 38.

Song, J. H., Shin, W. S., Yeoun, P. S., Choi, M. D. (2009). The influence of forest therapeutic program on unmarried mother's depression and self-esteem. *Journal of the Korean Forestry Society, 98*(1), 82–87.

Thoma, M. V., La Marca, R., Brönnimann, R., Finkel, L., Ehlert, U., & Nater, U. M. (2013). The effect of music on the human stress response. *PloS One, 8*(8), e70156.

Ulrich, R. S. (1983). Aesthetic and affective response to natural environments. In I. Altman & J. F. Wohlwill (Eds.), *Human behavior and the environment* (pp. 85–125). New York, NY: Plenum Press.

Ulrich, R. S. (1993). Biophilia, biophobia, and natural landscapes. In S. R. Kellert & E. O. Wilson (Eds.), *The biophilia hypothesis.* Washington, DC: Island Press/Shearwater.

Ulrich, R. S., Robert, F. S., Barbara, D. L., Evelyn, F., Mark, A. M., & Michael, Z. (1991). Stress recovery during exposure to natural and urban environments. *Journal of Environmental Psychology, 11*(3), 201–230.

You, Y. S., Kim, H. C., Lee, C. J., Jang, N. C., & Son, B. K. (2014). A study of effects of forest therapy-based mental health program on depression and psychological stability. *The Journal of Korean Society for School & Community Health Education, 15*(3), 55–65.

Wu, Z., Wang, C., Xu, J., & Hu, L. X. (2007). Air-borne anions and particulate matter in six urban green spaces during the summer. *Journal – Tsinghua University, 47*(12), 2153.

Part III

Critical Perspectives and Conclusions

Chapter 14

Critical Perspectives on Outdoor Therapy Practices

Denise Mitten

As introduced throughout this book, the type and diversity of outdoor therapies continues to grow. The aim of this chapter is to critically examine some basic assumptions about theory and practice underpinning the implementation of outdoor therapies. To do so, I examine the stories and histories that have been told about the roots of outdoor therapies, biased language, and relationships with the outdoors or nature. Most therapies are premised on the acts of beneficence (to do good) and nonmaleficence (to do no harm). However, sometimes practitioners have internalized assumptions, beliefs, and biases that may be harmful to people or certain populations. In fact, sometimes facilitators may assume beneficence, and might not recognize their actions or behavior as offending or harmful (Ansara & Hegarty, 2014). My goal is to offer readers tools and concepts to use as they design, build, and evaluate outdoor therapy programs and practices, and to inform future conversations and learning for practice.

The Author's Perspective

I am a woman residing in the United States who is involved in promoting health and well-being as well as teaching ecopsychology, sustainability education, outdoor/adventure education, and leadership. I highly value service, the ethic of care, and social justice for humans and the more-than-human worlds. I identify as a feminist/ecofeminist as well as a scholar-practitioner. My relationship with the natural world is heavily influenced by a childhood outdoors and my study of ecology and trees (forestry). Systems and complexity theory (Meadows, 2008) were part of my 1970s forestry education, which helps me see the world and relationships more from an ecological view than a hierarchical view. I have further training in parent education, complementary and alternative medicine, counseling, and outdoor leadership, through which I have developed a transdisciplinary lens to use in life and teaching. I consider the natural environment/more-than-human world my mentor. I believe the healing power of nature—expanded to the cosmos—has been overlooked and undervalued by many health practitioners, city and community planners, school personnel, parents, and even outdoor educators (Itin & Mitten, 2009; Mitten 2004). I and others have proposed that a major contributing factor to the global changes participants/clients experience after outdoor adventure programs/interventions, including adventure therapy and other outdoor therapies, may be the impact of being in and with the natural environment (Bardwell, 1992; Beringer & Martin, 2003; Mitten, 1994); in short, less about *doing*, and more about *being* (Mitten, 2004).

Critical Thinking

I critique because heritage gives us both wisdom from the past and shackles that must be shed to develop practices that benefit from the experience, research, and intuitive work done by a diversity of people (Fisher; 2019; Harper, Gabrielsen, & Carpenter, 2018; Itin & Mitten, 2009; Mitten, 1994; Nicholls & Gray, 2009; Warren, Roberts, Breunig, & Alvarez, 2014; Yamada, & San Antonio, 2009). Through fair-minded critique, practitioners and researchers can be more aware of and evaluate the strengths of outdoor therapies as well as harmful practices that may persist (Paul & Elder, 2016).

Critical thinking, which looks deeply at a subject or process, uses a questioning approach that, in a sense, never ends, and when used well, leads to continuously increasing understanding and a move toward overcoming egocentrism and socio-centrism (Paul & Elder, 2016). A critical approach includes how to deconstruct our beliefs using and assessing the quality of our thinking based on an intent to be fair. That is because the use of critical thinking helps people be aware of their preconceptions, prejudices, and biases. When I critique, my goal is to question with curiosity and purpose.

As an example, the concept of *best practices*, first recorded in use in 1927 and defined as a procedure that has been shown by research and experience to produce optimal results (Merriam Webster, 2019) can be examined critically. Because people practicing in outdoor therapies are well intended, there is a drive to identify practices that effectively help clients. Best practice is a word that many people innocently use to try to identify what methods and techniques to employ. Best practices can, however, stall critical thinking and influence people to stop innovating. If we have the best, there is none better. If we already have decided this is the best practice, then why critique it? Best practices are often represented as the most efficient and prudent way of doing something; with that in mind, if there is a best practice, it may imply, correctly or not, that one size fits all and essentializes people.

The concept of best practices represents Cartesian thought where it is assumed that through a linear progression of research we can get to *the truth* or the one best or right way of doing something, and, that there is a one way of doing something that works for all populations or situations (Bowers, 2007). This is problematic without acknowledging that the direction of research is influenced by political, social, and economic motives and interest of the researchers, sponsoring institutions, and research funders (Harding, 2015). Research produced within frameworks of the dominant groups (e.g., social, economic, racial, etc.) then form social policy and best practices for everyone to follow. One could call for research to be conducted using diverse populations, though that does not address the problem of limited methodologies and bias assumptions of Cartesian thought (Harding, 2015). Cartesian thinking is troubling because it reinforces *cultural hegemony* (cultural perspectives formed through everyday practices and shared beliefs become skewed in favor of the dominant group and provide the foundation for complex systems of domination) and does not recognize discontinuity of an idea (Bowers, 2007) or *cultural discontinuity*, lack of consistency between two or more cultures (Cholewa & West-Olatunji, 2008; Ogbu, 1982). Cultural hegemony of the dominant group is maintained, in part, through championing best practices. In outdoor therapies, the dominant culture has more access to publishing (Martin, Maney, & Mitten, 2018) and therefore in creating, articulating, and maintaining best practices.

As an example, a common practice in many outdoor therapies is asking or telling people to get out of, or expand, their *comfort zone*. Leaders are making an assumption, even if unconsciously, that the person is comfortable, even if one says it as a euphemism. Boilen (2018) explored the psychological and relational implications of participation in an intentionally unfamiliar excursion. Participants literally step out of their familiar realms and have opportunities to be in an unfamiliar situation and try on new and unfamiliar behaviors. In this case, they are leaving their familiar, not their comfort. To ask a military veteran living with post-traumatic stress disorder, a youth living on the street, a person in prison, or even a high school student with anxiety to get out of their comfort zone may be disrespectful, and, though well intended, probably comes from a privileged place on the leader's part. The comfort zone concept is likely an artifact from the early days of outdoor and adventure education when the thought was that young people were getting too soft and needed to toughen up!

Another practice often labeled a best practice and commonly used in many outdoor therapy programs is a concept called *challenge by choice*. The effects of challenge by choice have not been well researched. Tyson and Asmus (2008) argued that the challenge by choice paradigm may not offer authentic choice that is central to an experience of personal empowerment. They pointed out three concerns for participants being able to make authentic choices using challenge by choice: (1) the underlying values of the facilitator and/or program often create a culture that rewards only certain choices, (2) practitioners often see their role as moving individuals toward a desired outcome, which compromises choice, and (3) many participants in outdoor programs may lack the support and education to make healthy choices. Haras, Bunting, and Witt (2006) described a model, *inviting optimum participation,* for ropes course programs that includes a wide range of clearly defined ways to be involved in the activities. Comparing that model with challenge by choice, their research found the optimum participation approach elicited lower levels of anxiety, and a higher degree of perceived choice and similar degrees of meaningful involvement. Supporting participant choice and shared decision-making can be employed without using challenge by choice by implementing program components such as providing participants with options, having flexible schedules, allowing people their own timing, encouraging rather than pushing, giving participants information to make informed choices, and intentionally supporting individuals in defining and making choices for themselves (Mitten, 1985).

What Stories Are Told about the Roots of Outdoor Therapies?

The current dominant history of outdoor therapies, as found in web searches, seems to have a great deal of agreement. Most versions place the origin in the United States in the 1800s with tent camps for tuberculosis patients, highlighting that outdoor therapy is not a new concept. They talk about the therapeutic camp movement in the early 1900s and experiential education. Two individuals named most often (and frequently the only two mentioned) are educators John Dewey and Kurt Hahn. These selective pieces make this history mostly American and European male-centric, and frame it through the camping and adventure movement, importing many assumptions in practice from these fields. Some theorists and researchers have tried to broaden outdoor therapies histories (e.g., Cole, Erdman, & Rothblum, 1994; Gray & Mitten, 2018; Mitten, Gray, Allen-Craig, Loeffler, & Carpenter, 2018; Richards, 2003) and practitioners have been encouraged to critically examine histories of their specific modality.

There is rarely one right history about anything. Often there are certain facts, such as people who were involved or events that happened that are accurate. However, usually more people were involved, and many more events happened than are represented. But when a subset of events and people are repeated in many stories, they become the conventional history that informs practice. For example, it is commonly thought that Kurt Hahn invented the adventure education expedition model, though it was discovered that Marina Ewald, a geographer, was a key player and instrumental to the inception of the Outward Bound expeditionary model (Veevers & Allison, 2011). Ewald initiated the school's first sailing expedition to Finland and Iceland in 1925. As a result of her advocacy for expeditions in the curriculum, Hahn embedded them into Outward Bound. After Hahn left Germany, Ewald directed Salem school for another 50 years.

Often these histories are translated into writing and practices are called traditions, for example, "traditionally outdoor therapies have used challenge by choice." Using the word traditional makes it sound vetted or well established. Appropriate questions would challenge practices to show what research they are based on, which populations they are appropriate for, and for what purpose(s). Ultimately, is it an appropriate practice for the population with whom I work, the programming I use, and the desired client outcomes?

Other authors have questioned the use of stress as a learning tool in outdoor therapies (Berman & Davis-Berman, 2005; Mitten, 1986). Jensen and Simovka (2005) advocated that learning environments do not rely on stress because he found that students under stress are less able to understand connections, and that when stressed, the brain tends not to use highest order cognitive function (e.g., careful and critical thinking). Also, research supports that people, for example, recovering from breast cancer who engaged in outdoor restorative activities reported quality of life improvement when participating in relaxing non-stressful activities (Cimprich, 1993).

A number of outdoor therapies described in this book do not use risk and stress as primary program components, such as ecopsychology and forest therapy. Bardwell (1992) reinforced this approach when she reported on a study about a program modeled after the Outward Bound program, with one distinct difference: The program did not include many of the stresses and challenges of a typical Outward Bound course. The results showed similar global changes in client behaviors and attitudes as reports from the programs with more stress and challenge. Bottomline is that stress, risk, and challenge require more research as to their utility in programming in outdoor therapies.

Risk is complicated, and means different things to different people, and what feels risky is an individual experience. Risk can be fun and rewarding, yet risk aversion (though not to a maladapted level) in many areas is healthy (e.g., fear of snakes, heights). Risk can be addictive, such as in gambling or wanting to have adrenaline rushes, and risk can help some people feel powerful and superior (Mitten & Whittingham, 2009). Positively, in risky situations, with appropriate facilitation, participants can develop the ability to understand and work with fear appropriately and they can develop the ability to manage cognitions and emotions under stress. Purposefully taking risks to prove competency for courage is different than gaining competency through skill development and participating meaningfully in adventures that may involve risk.

Hyping perceived risk has been observed in some outdoor therapy marketing materials and is a deception that may inhibit teaching wise judgment about risk and risk-taking behaviors. Instead of learning judgment about which risks to take, with whom to take them, when not to take them, and how to use judgment to decide between factors, participants may learn that risk taking in itself is the positive action and leave the program thinking that if they do not choose risk they are not courageous. Or, they might leave the program and not make the outdoors part of their lives because they did not embrace the exhilaration they were told comes with risk taking. Practitioners in outdoor therapies are encouraged to pay attention to the attributes around the risk-taking rather than the risky action in itself.

Trade a Paternal Historical Lens for an Ecological One

A way to help transform a narrow and select memory of history is to counter the Western tradition of ownership, including paternal inheritance. The practice of believing there are founders, usually founding 'fathers,' decreases inclusion, reinforces a hierarchy, and contributes to the dominance of primarily white men and the marginalization of others. For example, the orthodox lineage in the literature of experiential education, and by extension some outdoor therapies—Socrates, Plato, Aristotle, Hahn, and Dewey—is exclusively 'fathers' (Wurdinger, 1997). Perhaps it is time to shed the parental metaphor, which reinforces a gender binary and heterosexualization (Mitten, 2013), which in turn reinforces biological determinism of outdoor and environmental education, including some outdoor therapies (Russell, Sarick, & Kennelly, 2002). Mitten (2013) suggested changing the conversation from a genealogical point of view to that of an ecological system, emphasizing that people from a number of intellectual and practical niches have contributed to outdoor therapies from their perspectives in their respective areas. A different paradigm—that of ecology and relationships, for example— can uncover more of the richness of outdoor therapies, and encourage greater participation and creativity. Thinking in terms of systems and relationships encourages people to look in a variety of niches to find complementary contributions and question dominant paradigms. A systems perspective may help open peoples' capacities to value and include more works of women and other underrepresented groups in scholarly discussions about outdoor therapies.

In an ecological system, seemingly small contributions may be crucial for the whole ecosystem to thrive. Piersol and Timmerman (2017) reinforced a paradigm of an ecology of relationships by using a lived ecofeminist politic to engage more voices and diversity and redistribute power in academia. Tuck, McKenzie, and McCoy (2014) and Root (2010) discussed the need to *decolonize* (heal from the forces of colonialism) outdoor and environmental education, which can be extended to outdoor therapies (Fisher, 2019). Jones and Segal (2018), non-Indigenous/settler practitioners, specifically called for unsettling ecopsychology by deep reflection by practitioners to encourage "accountability for those doing therapeutic land-based nature connection work as visitors on traditional Indigenous territories" (p. 1). These authors make the argument that ecopsychology practices can reproduce and reinforce settler colonialism. Among other things, using an ecological and systems perspective when talking about contributions to the field can contribute to diversifying and the decentering of white European practices and thinking in outdoor therapies.

Instead of situating outdoor therapies as beginning in the last couple of centuries, practitioners might learn more by conceiving of the reciprocal relationship between humans and the more-than-human worlds that has been interdependent and persisted since the evolution of humans six million years ago (Flinders, 2003). In a sense, outdoor therapies are modalities that can strengthen the healthy connections or relationships between humans and the more-than-human world—connections that are still strong, though often estranged in many societies.

How a facilitator and the modality relate to the outdoor environment, and how a practitioner encourages clients to relate to nature are key considerations for outdoor therapy practitioners. For some, nature is a partner in the treatment. Other practitioners talk about using nature to aid in healing or recovery. Still others create awe around the *divine feminine* (life energy) or creation that is nature and the cosmos. Attitudes and beliefs around the natural environment influence practice and some practices may be vulnerable to colonizing values (Fisher, 2019). For example, through language and practice, intentional or not, nature is often:

- seen as something from which humans are disconnected;
- seen as separate from culture and in a binary with culture;
- viewed as a commodity or used to feel better;
- dominated and used to prove competency or power; and
- anthropomorphized.

Studies show that in the United States at least 38% of girls and 24% of boys have been sexually abused by the time they are 18 by someone designated as a caregiver, meaning that on outdoor therapy programs, even those not designated for survivors, one in three women and one in seven men may have been abused (Smith et al., 2017). For survivors of sexual abuse, "interaction with certain natural elements such as flies and mosquitoes, rain and lightning, dirt, and darkness can trigger sexual abuse memories and feelings, and even panic" (Mitten & Dutton, 1993, p. 135). Working with natural elements out of one's control or an inability to clean oneself like at home can be challenging for many people and more so for certain populations. Though some programs have used trauma-informed care at least since the 1970s, this is becoming more common on many programs, causing it to be susceptible to be singularly defined and implemented. Some practitioners might believe that nature's effects are distributed impartially. However, coming to an outdoor program afraid of nature might indicate a need for gentle introductions to nature rather than immediate deep immersion and a model of programming that does not attend to individual differences.

Being able to be comfortable in a facilitated group in nature means being able to feel safe being oneself and safe trying on new roles (at the individual's pace). As practitioners we may know little about our participants. Many people rely on a visual read of participants' identities for race/ethnicity, able-bodiedness, age, and gender—often using the binary lens of female and male to assign participants' gender identities. Some practitioners may misread or 'misgender' client identities, committing what Ansara and Hegarty (2014) call 'cisgenderism' (p. 260). This practice can erase non-binary identities. People can identify and express gender in a multiplicity of ways including but not limited to women, men, persons with non-binary gender identities, agender, gender-queer, gender non-conforming, transgender, and intersex individuals (Ansara & Hegarty, 2014). An inclusivity solution is not necessarily obvious. Some practitioners have instituted a practice of having clients say their preferred pronouns, which for some clients can be uncomfortable coming out so soon in a new group of people (or they are questioning) and feel put on the spot at having to respond. Being inclusive is a process without a well-defined path. From marketing materials to the close of the program messages go out about who is welcome on the program. A practitioner's experience, education, and reflexivity aid in creating space and pace for participants to establish healthy relationships.

Human and Nature Attachment: A Rethink on Pathology

In addition to *time* in nature, the *kind* of relationship established with nature through outdoor therapies is a crucial consideration. Human physical proximity may be removed from natural environments because so much time is spent in built environments, however, humans are part of the living system of earth and, quite literally, humans cannot disconnect from nature. The notion of diagnosing nature-disconnect or 'nature-deficit' smacks of pathologizing and the medical model of treatment (Harper, Rose, & Segal, 2019). Rather, many humans likely have a disordered attachment, and an estranged relationship with nature (Mitten, 2017).

Young people may have insecure attachments to a caregiver, signs of which commonly include lack of impulse control, violence, and tendency toward addictions as well as anxiety, depression, and difficulty in emotional regulation (Fairchild, 2006). The notion of a disordered attachment with nature has similar symptoms for a great many people in Western culture, including many of those who may come to experience healing in outdoor therapies. A healthy attachment with nature can help people in similar ways that healthy human attachment does, including feeling secure, having the ability to seek out social support (as well as time in nature for support), share feelings with other people, enter into trusting relationships, and enjoy intimate relationships (D'Amore & Mitten, 2015). Rather than seeing clients with diagnoses, we might also consider how attached or disconnected one is from nature. This perspective shift may allow for positive benefits to accrue in our client's lives that become ongoing resources for them outside of therapy such as visiting a local beach or forest to recover from daily stress (Mitten, Overholt, Haynes, D'Amore, & Ady, 2016).

A useful question for practitioners to ask is what kind of attachment with nature am I encouraging or reinforcing? A relationship based on mutualism, respect, and curiosity may be more beneficial for holistic healing than a relationship based on using nature or dominating it (e.g., nature as resource or conquering a mountain). A practitioner's modeling and encouragement about relationships can help foster these mutual relationships and discourage domination relationships. Outdoor therapies can be incubators of learning about and experiencing healthy relationships with nature. Thoughtfully designed outdoor therapies with leaders skilled in healthy relationship building have the potential to provide rich, transformative, paradigm shifting experiences for their participants.

Conclusion

This critique offered several concepts and common assumptions about outdoor therapies, and leaves many questions for practitioners to ask of themselves and their work. What stories have been used to build the history and body of knowledge commonly used in outdoor therapies and what perhaps differing stories are out there? Where do we practice and are we sensitive to the lands on which our services and programs are offered? Do the 'traditions' of outdoor therapies rely on assumptions of doing good, or are they possibly causing harm? Language is central in the development of ethical client engagement, drives practice, and has huge impacts on outcomes.

One way to ensure we maintain ethical and moral perspectives toward our services and our clients is to continually critique our theory and practice. There are, obviously, many more ethical questions that need to be examined regarding outdoor therapies and I hope that this chapter helps practitioners and researchers in outdoor therapies to shine a critical light on our work to ensure the positive outcomes and care for all clients.

References

Ansara, Y. G. & Hegarty, P. (2014). Methodologies of misgendering: Recommendations for reducing cisgenderism in psychological research. *Feminism & Psychology, 24*(2), 259–270. doi:10.1177/0959353514526217

Bardwell, L. (1992). A bigger piece of the puzzle: The restorative experience and outdoor education. In Henderson (Ed.), *Coalition for education in the outdoors: Research symposium proceeding* (pp. 15–20). Bradford Woods, IN: Coalition for Education in the Outdoors.

Beringer, A. & Martin. P. (2003). On adventure therapy and the natural worlds: Respecting nature's healing. *Journal of Adventure Education & Outdoor Learning, 3*(1), 29–39.

Berman, D. S. & Davis-Berman, J. (2005). Positive psychology and outdoor education. *Journal of Experiential Education, 28*(1), 17–24.

Boilen, S. (2018). The backcountry of the female mind: Young women's voices from the wilderness. In T. Gray & D. Mitten (Eds.), *The Palgrave international handbook of women and outdoor learning* (pp. 449–460). Cham, Switzerland: Palgrave Macmillan.

Bowers, C. A. (2007). Philosophy, language, and the Titanic mind-set. *Language and Ecology, 2*(2), 1–15.

Cholewa, B. & West-Olatunji, C. (2008). Exploring the relationship among cultural discontinuity, psychological distress, and academic outcomes with low-income, culturally diverse students. *Professional School Counseling, 12*(1), 2156759X0801200106.

Cimprich, B. (1993). Development of an intervention to restore attention in cancer patients. *Cancer Nursing, 16*(2), 83–92.

Cole, E., Erdman, E, &. Rothblum, E. (Eds.) (1994). *Wilderness therapy for women: The power of adventure*. Binghamton, NY: Harrington Press.

D'Amore, C. & Mitten, D. (2015). Nurtured nature: The connection between care for children and care for the environment. In P. L. Thomas, P. Carr, J. Gorlewski, & B. Porfilio (Eds.), *Pedagogies of kindness and respect: On the lives and education of children* (pp. 111–125). New York, NY: Peter Lang.

Fairchild, S. R. (2006). Understanding attachment: Reliability and validity of selected attachment measures for preschoolers and children. *Child and Adolescent Social Work Journal, 23*(2), 235–261.

Fisher, A. (2019). Ecopsychology as decolonial praxis. *Ecopsychology, 11*(3), 145–155.

Flinders, C. (2003). *Rebalancing the world: Why women belong and men compete and how to restore the ancient equilibrium.* San Francisco, CA: HarperCollins.

Gray, T. & Mitten, D. (Eds.) (2018). *The Palgrave international handbook of women and outdoor learning.* Cham, Switzerland: Palgrave MacMillan.

Haras, K., Bunting, C., & Witt, P. (2006). Meaningful involvement opportunities in ropes course programs. *Journal of Leisure Research, 38*(3), 339–363.

Harding, S. (2015). *Objectivity and diversity: Another logic of scientific research.* University of Chicago Press.

Harper, N. J., Gabrielsen, L. E., & Carpenter, C. (2018). A cross-cultural exploration of 'wild' in wilderness therapy: Canada, Norway and Australia. *Journal of Adventure Education and Outdoor Learning, 18*(2), 148–164.

Harper, N., Rose, K., & Segal, D. (2019). *Nature base therapy: A practitioner's guide to working with children, youth and families.* Gabriola Island, BC: New Society Publishers.

Itin, C. & Mitten, D. (2009). The nature and meaning of adventure therapy in the international context. In D. Mitten & C. M. Itin (Eds.), *Connecting with the essence of adventure therapy: Proceedings from the 4th international adventure therapy conference (2006)* (pp. 5–12). Boulder, CO: Association for Experiential Education.

Jensen, B. B., & Simovska, V. (2005). Involving students in learning and health promotion processes: Clarifying why? What? And how?. *Promotion & Education, 12*(3), 150–156.

Jones, A. T. & Segal, D. S. (2018). Unsettling ecopsychology: Addressing settler colonialism in ecopsychology practice. *Ecopsychology, 10*(3), 127–136.

Martin, S., Maney, S., & Mitten, D. (2018). Messages about women through representation in adventure education texts and journals. In T. Gray & D. Mitten (Eds.), *The Palgrave international handbook of women and outdoor learning* (pp. 293–306). Palgrave Macmillan.

Meadows, D. H. (2008). *Thinking in systems: A primer.* Hartford, VT: Chelsea Green Publishing.

Merriam Webster Dictionary. (2019). Retrieved June 19, 2019 from https://www.merriam-webster.com/dictionary/best%20practice

Mitten, D. (1985). A philosophical basis for a women's outdoor adventure program. *Journal of Experiential Education, 8*(2), 20–24.

Mitten, D. (1986). Stress management and wilderness activities. In M. Gass & L. Buel (Eds.), *Proceedings journal.* Moodus, CT: Association of Experiential Education 14th Annual Conference.

Mitten, D., & Dutton, R. (1993). Outdoor leadership considerations with women survivors of sexual abuse. *Journal of Experiential Education, 16*(1), 7–13.

Mitten, D. (1994). Ethical considerations in adventure therapy: A feminist critique. In E. Cole, E. Erdman, & E. Rothblum (Eds.), *Wilderness therapy for women: The power of adventure* (pp. 55–84). Binghamton, NY: Harrington Press.

Mitten, D. (2004). Adventure therapy as complementary and alternative therapy. In S. Bandoroff & S. Newes (Eds.), *Coming of Age: The evolving field of adventure therapy* (pp. 240–257). Boulder, CO: Association of Experiential Education.

Mitten, D. & Whittingham, M. (2009). Be safe out there: Critically thinking risk in adventure education. In B. Stremba & C. Bisson (Eds.), *Teaching adventure education theory best practices*. Champaign, IL: Human Kinetics.

Mitten, D. (2013). Book review: Sourcebook of experiential education: Key thinkers and their contributions. *Journal of Experiential Education, 36*(1), 80–82.

Mitten, D., Overholt, J. R., Haynes, F. I., D'Amore, C. C., & Ady, J. C. (2016). Hiking. A low-cost, accessible intervention to promote health benefits. *American Journal of Lifestyle Medicine, 12*(4), 302–310.

Mitten, D. (2017). Connections, compassion, and co-healing: The ecology of relationship. In K. Malone, S. Truong, & T. Gray (Eds.), *Reimagining sustainability in precarious times* (pp. 173–186). London, England: Springer.

Mitten, D., Gray, T., Allen-Craig, S., Loeffler, T. A., & Carpenter, C. (2018). The invisibility cloak: Women's contributions to outdoor and environmental education. *The Journal of Environmental Education, 49*(4), 318–327.

Nicholls, V. & Gray, T. (2009). Sense and sensibility: Reality and romanticism in human/nature relationships. In D. Mitten & C. M. Itin (Eds.), *Connecting with the essence of adventure therapy: Proceedings from the 4th international adventure therapy conference (2006)* (pp. 158–168). Boulder, CO: Association for Experiential Education.

Ogbu, J. U. (1982). Cultural discontinuities and schooling. *Anthropology & Education Quarterly, 13*(4), 290–307.

Paul, R. & Elder, L. (2016). *The miniature guide to critical thinking concepts & tools*. Lanham, MD: Rowman & Littlefield Publishers.

Piersol, L. & Timmerman, N. (2017). Reimagining environmental education within academia: Storytelling and dialogue as lived ecofeminist politics. *The Journal of Environmental Education, 48*(1), 10–17.

Richards, K. (2003). Critical feminist reflexive research in adventure therapy and eating disorders: Exposing the narrative (s) of a relational, embodied and gendered self. In B. Humberstone, H. Brown, & K. Richards (Eds.), *Whose Journeys? The Outdoors and Adventure as Social and Cultural Phenomena* (pp. 49–74). Barrow-in-Furness, England: Fingerprints.

Root, E. (2010). This land is our land? This land is your land: The decolonizing journeys of white outdoor environmental educators. *Canadian Journal of Environmental Education, 15*, 103–119.

Russell, C. L., Sarick, T., & Kennelly, J. (2002). Queering environmental education. *Canadian Journal of Environmental Education, 7*(1), 54–66.

Smith, S. G., Chen, J., Basile, K. C., Gilbert, L. K., Merrick, M. T., Patel, N., ..., Jain, A. (2017). The National Intimate Partner and Sexual Violence Survey (NISVS): 2010–2012 state report. Retrieved from the Centers for Disease Control and Prevention, National Center for Injury Prevention and Control, https://www.cdc.gov/violenceprevention/pdf/NISVS-StateReportBook.pdf

Tuck, E., McKenzie, M., & McCoy, K. (2014). Land education: Indigenous, post-colonial, and decolonizing perspectives on place and environmental education research. *Environmental Education Research, 20*(1), 1–23.

Tyson, L. & Asmus, K. (2008). Deepening the paradigm of choice: Exploring choice and power in experiential education. In K. Warren, D. Mitten, & T. A. Loeffler (Eds.), *Theory and practice of experiential education*. Association for Experiential education.

Veevers, N. & Allison, P. (2011). *Kurt Hahn*. Rotterdam, Netherlands: Sense Publishers.

Warren, K., Roberts, N. S., Breunig, M., & Alvarez, M. A. G. (2014). Social justice in outdoor experiential education: A state of knowledge review. *Journal of Experiential Education*, 37(1), 89–103.

Wurdinger, S. D. (1997). *Philosophical issues in adventure education*. Dubuque, IA: Kendall Hunt.

Yamada, S. & San Antonio, D. (2009). Toward a common understanding: A method for organizing terminology in the field of adventure therapy. In D. Mitten & C. M. Itin (Eds.), *Connecting with the essence of adventure therapy: Proceedings from the 4th international adventure therapy conference* (pp. 180–198). Boulder, CO: Association for Experiential Education.

Chapter 15

Future Direction for Outdoor Therapies

Will W. Dobud and Daniel L. Cavanaugh

Introduction

Over the past half-century, there has been a significant increase in literature, awareness, and research encouraging helping professionals to take therapy outdoors. Texts such as Gass, Gillis, and Russell's (2012) comprehensive discussion of adventure therapy and Harper, Rose, and Segal's (2019) practical discussion of nature-based therapy are just three works which demonstrate the considerable effort to raise the credibility and recognition of outdoor therapies. Further, accessible texts such as Williams' (2017) *The Nature Fix* and Selhub and Logan's (2012) *Your Brain on Nature*, have sold the biological, psychological, and physiological benefits of spending time in natural environments and have rose in popularity.

What has been missing is a collection and exploration of numerous yet distinct allied approaches as is included in this book. Outdoor therapies, such as wilderness therapy, have been criticized for being too varied and poorly defined to stand a chance against the bona-fide psychotherapies, such as cognitive behavioral or psychodynamic therapy (Becker & Russell, 2016). The lack of a coherent theory of change also means questioning the active ingredients for each of these models (Dobud & Harper, 2018), as Carpenter and Pryor explored in Chapter 7. The quality of research, some questionable ethics, and a lack of professionalism have certainly challenged the history and popularity of this particular outdoor therapy which we practice and advocate for (Dobud, Cavanaugh, & Harper, 2020; Harper, 2017).

Given the global contributions of scholars and practitioners, and the span of outdoor therapy approaches—from surfing to horticulture and wilderness to animal-assisted—this book provides a detailed overview of the current status of the diverse field of outdoor therapies. Having examined the chapters, we feel comfortable, although humble as two emerging academics, to present some of the key themes from the text and to critically discuss future directions for the field.

A Synopsis of the Outdoor Therapies

Providing a brief synopsis of what occurred in this book was challenging. There are many unique perspectives, which might simply be showcasing the range of outdoor therapy practice and perspectives informing this work. The contributing chapters covered a range of professions; social work, psychology, counselling, family therapy, occupational therapy, to name a few. After all, many of the chapters mentioned that their contribution to this book is just one approach to their work. For example, wilderness therapy in the Scandinavian approach is described a different mode of wilderness therapy, though described with the same terminology, than in the United States (see Chapter 6). Though diversity is something we honor, this can potentially confuse researchers and service users. In this case, we urge practitioners of outdoor therapies to understand, articulate, and promote their models and values clearly.

While reviewing these chapters, we paid particular attention to the available literature and evidence. Many authors noted the boundaries of their knowledge base, such as the limitations of how nature-based therapy transcends cultural preferences, locations, and populations (see Chapter 8). Notwithstanding these limitations, we wish to pronounce an important conclusion about taking therapy into the outdoors: *it works*. Meta-analyses and systematic reviews (e.g., Bowen & Neill, 2013) have provided considerable evidence to suggest these modalities are effective ways for therapists to approach working with their clients. Based on this introductory text, we can see the potential for these outdoor therapies as the body of evidence supporting these practices develop. That said, we did locate areas worthy of future consideration, including a lack of client voice and preventative programs, which are explored in the following sections.

Client Voice

In comparison to many older conventional talk therapies, such as psychoanalytic therapy, outdoor therapy literature seems to grow and develop each decade (Harper, 2017). Advocates of different approaches have worked tirelessly to produce strong empirical evidence that these outdoor approaches really work. Large-scale meta-analyses including thousands of participants have demonstrated the effects of outdoor therapies (Annerstedt & Währborg, 2011; Bettmann, Gillis, Speelman, Parry, & Case, 2016; Bowen & Neill, 2013; Gillis et al., 2016). However, what is still largely absent from the outdoor therapy literature is a thorough qualitative exploration of client's perspectives on what it is like to participate in outdoor therapies.

Recent Google Scholar searches that combined terms such as "adventure therapy," "nature-based therapies," and "outdoor therapies" with the terms "client-voice," "participant voice," "client perspectives," and "participant perspectives" all returned less than ten results each. In contrast, a search that combined "client perspectives" with "psychotherapy" returned 2,300 results. Scholars, such as Bell (2015), have described the need to incorporate youth voice into mental health and psychotherapy literature. It is time for outdoor therapies to heed this call and begin to find ways to include the voice of our clients in our research and program development.

Despite an overall shortage of research including client voice and perspectives, a handful of studies have emerged to explore the voices of clients who have participated in different outdoor programs. These studies can be used as exemplars for the creation of future research that includes the voices of those we serve. Promising work by Harper, Mott, and Obee (2019) explored the perspectives of 138 young people who participated in a Canadian outdoor therapy program describing improved health, changes in self-concept, skills developed, social dynamics, the outdoor setting, and what the youth perceived as catalysts for change. Dobud (2020) conducted interviews and participant observation with young people who participated in adventure therapy programs around the world. These young people described a variety of experiences. Some of them have described challenging, even traumatic experiences, in wilderness therapy. Others reported positive experiences, such as mastering outdoor skills, self-discovery, and describing in-depth some ideas about beneficial therapeutic relationships in outdoor therapy settings.

While many of the authors in this book described the physical, emotional, and psychological benefits of participating in outdoor therapy, their case vignettes accentuated how the context of what brings a client to therapy, the interpersonal skills of the therapist, and the quality of their relationship, which includes consensus about the purpose of their work together, was essential to the success of the therapy. Future qualitative research should explore client perspectives on what they believe helped or hindered their progress in outdoor therapies or explore what helped to consolidate therapeutic gains post-intervention.

Prevention

Outdoor prevention programs were an area we noticed lacking throughout this book. From our review, we noticed brief references to the opportunity for approaching this work from a preventative approach. In Chapter 6, Fernee and Gabrielsen mentioned the use of wilderness therapy as a preventative measure in school settings. Chapter 13, Shin and Lee presented how forest therapy can be delivered as a preventative approach and Ponting, in Chapter 12, described prevention in the International Surf Therapy Organization's (2019) definition of surf therapy, which they referred to as "a therapeutic vehicle in the prevention and treatment of social, behavioral, health, economic, and other challenges" (n.p.). Given our interest in prevention, particularly based on the second author's research interests and participation in two international research collaborations, one focused on prevention (Riebschleger, Costello, Cavanaugh, & Grové, 2019; Riebschleger, Grové, Costello, & Cavanaugh, 2018) and the other on adventure therapy (Dobud et al., 2020), we wished to provide discussion about the potential for a preventative focus in outdoor therapies.

Young people today face an array of increased behavioral health risks related to or including: mental illness, substance abuse, bullying, criminal justice involvement, behavioral challenges, and suicide/self-harm (Burke, Hellman, Scott, Weems, & Carrion, 2011; Hawton, Saunders, & O'Connor, 2012; Merikangas & McClair, 2012; Modecki, Minchin, Harbaugh, Guerra, & Runions, 2014; Steel et al., 2014). Young people who have experienced traumatic events, referred to as adverse childhood experiences, face increased risks of future mental illness as well as physical health maladies, such as diabetes or heart problems (Dube, Anda, Felitti, Edwards, & Croft, 2002; Monnat & Chandler, 2015; Schilling, Aseltine, & Gore, 2007). These risks are further exacerbated by the challenges of living in a world facing mass environmental degradation and global warming, which may lead to further behavioral challenges (Scull, 2008). Challenging times call for the need to offer preventative programming that can keep people from needing additional treatment later in their lives.

Effective prevention interventions include a range of psychoeducation, social support, community support, and coping skill development programs (Masten, 2014; Kutcher, Bagnell, & Wei, 2015). Additionally, researchers have learned that time in natural environments may promote resiliency and prevent mental illness (Annerstedt & Währborg, 2011). A small subset of this field has begun to emerge that is using techniques from adventure therapy and other outdoor interventions to combine the benefits of time in natural environments with prevention programming to counter the increased behavioral health risks faced by young people today (Beightol, Jevertson, Carter, Gray, & Gass, 2012; Carter, Straits, & Hall, 2007; Ritchie, Wabano, Russell, Enosse, & Young, 2014).

Two of the most well-documented examples of adventure-based prevention programming are from Project Venture and Santa Fe Mountain Center. These programs were recognized as evidence-based practices in the United States, by the National Registry of Evidence-Based Programs and Practices as evidence-based practices (Carter et al., 2007; Beightol et al., 2012). Project Venture's programming offers mountain biking, kayaking, camping, and other activities to Indigenous youth in the United States. They combine outdoor adventure activities with traditional Indigenous practices and tribal wisdom to develop resilience in the young people in their programs. At the Santa Fe Mountain Center, the Adventures in a Caring Community program fuses traditional prevention programming with activities, such as ropes courses, to foster resilience and relationship skills in school-aged young people. There are examples of programs around the world delivering preventative programs, such as Chicago Voyagers' work with inner city youth, the former Project Hahn's primary prevention program in Tasmania and New Zealand, and the Wikwemikong Outdoor Adventure Leadership Experience for Indigenous youth in Canada (Lan, Sveen, & Davidson, 2004; Ritchie et al., 2014). These programs are exemplars of how outdoor therapies can be used to not just treat behavioral health challenges, but to prevent them before they begin.

Focusing on the continuum of care and where outdoor therapies fit among other mental health approaches for behavioral risks raise important questions. Many authors suggested that taking therapy outside is beneficial when people have not benefited from conventional therapy. On the more extreme end, residential programming, common to wilderness therapy (e.g., Bettman et al., 2013), tends to work with young people who have experienced numerous treatment failures, leaving us with questions about how these outdoor approaches could become mainstream approaches for people with behavioral challenges, not just as a last resort. Ultimately, we became inspired by the level of advocacy and dedication from Won Sop Shin and Juyoung Lee in Chapter 13 and their discussion about getting forest therapy and its benefits recognized by the Korean federal government. Positioning the outdoor therapies as a mainstream option will take the same persistence as exemplified by those in Korea.

Embracing the Evidence: Implications for Future Research

The outcome research presented throughout this book has demonstrated an important and key finding: taking therapy outdoors works. Whether its adventure therapy (Bowen & Neill, 2013), wilderness therapy (Harper, 2017), or surf therapy (Michalewicz-Kragh, 2019), there is a scope of outcome studies supporting these diverse approaches. That said, we use this section as a call to action for outdoor therapy practitioners to embrace evidence, use it to inform their practice, and to build more of it themselves.

There are troubling findings relating to various models of therapy, client experiences in care, and therapist development. Since psychotherapy's first meta-analysis, conducted by Smith and Glass (1977), no differences in outcomes have emerged to suggest one mode of therapy is more effective than the next. In the last half century, this finding has become one of psychotherapy's most replicated findings, second only to the evidence that, yes, psychotherapy works and works well (Miller, Hubble, Chow, & Seidel, 2013). However, we now have over 600 types of therapy, including those listed in this book, but do not have the evidence to suggest any one is better than the next (Meichenbaum & Lilienfeld, 2018). Moreover, therapists tend to choose their preferred way of approaching clients based on personal values, not the available evidence (Caldwell, 2015). We, for example, acknowledge that our personal outdoor experiences led us to wanting to help others in outdoor environments. That said, scholars have raised concerns about this overcrowding of therapy models pointing us away from various model mania and urging us to look at individual therapist performance in, or out, of the counselling room (Dobud & Harper, 2018; Miller et al., 2013; Wampold & Imel, 2015). We present below some of these troubling yet illuminating studies from outside the outdoor therapies to inform our proposed agenda for future research and practice.

Hannan et al. (2005) conducted a study to see if therapists in a university clinic could accurately predict client dropout and deterioration on outcome measures. The therapists failed to identify 39 of the 40 clients reporting not to benefit from the psychotherapy services. Moreover, the largest and longest study of therapist development concluded that, on average, individual therapist outcomes decline with experience (Goldberg et al., 2016). This means that despite mandated continuing professional development, costly weekend workshops and conferences, or ongoing group or clinical supervision, it was a smaller percentage of practitioners who actually improved their performance with clients over time (Chow et al., 2015). Though taking therapy outside is nothing new, we can learn as a field how to avoid many of the same pitfalls, which are occurring in psychotherapy practice around the world (Caldwell, 2015). It begins by holding ourselves accountable in the outdoor therapies, as a diverse and experiential field, to implementing and informing our work based on the latest available evidence. This need was highlighted by Bowen and Neill (2013) who hypothesized that less than 1% of adventure therapy programs undergo any sort of program evaluation.

Most, if not all, of the psychotherapy professions push for practitioners to utilize the best available research when working with clients (Caldwell, 2015). As American social workers, we adhere to the National Association of Social Workers' (2017) code of ethics' standard 4.01 (c) which emphasizes that "Social workers should base practice knowledge on recognized knowledge, including empirically based knowledge, relevant to social work and social work ethics" (n.p.). If you are a counsellor or psychotherapist in Australia, your professional association has made public commitments to evidence-informed practice, maintaining that all its members "prioritise evidence-informed practice" and "the use of appropriate standardised outcome measures . . . to ensure that they received systematic feedback on the effectiveness of their services, and the systematic use of this feedback to improve practice" (PACFA, 2013, para. 4). Given the international scholarship within this text, we recommend readers look up their practice guidelines and ethical code of your profession (and in your region) to find statements such as these. We also urge practitioners of all theoretical orientations to embrace routine outcome monitoring as not only a fundamental component of their practice, but to build their own evidence (Dobud, 2017; Miller et al., 2013).

Though progress monitoring occurred as early as the 1960s, routine outcome monitoring was first championed by Howard et al. (1996), when the group of clinicians and researchers began systematically collecting outcome data before each therapy session. Researchers, such as Lambert et al. (2001), noticed the impact of outcome monitoring and found when outcome data was shared with practitioners about a client's progress in therapy, or lack thereof, client progress doubled, deterioration (or clients getting worse) decreased by 33%, and reduced the overall number of sessions attended by their clients.

There are now several meta-analyses and more than a dozen randomized clinical trials providing substantial evidence to support routine outcome monitoring in therapy (Miller, Hubble, Chow, & Seidel, 2015; Miller & Schuckard, 2014). We use outcome monitoring as an example for outdoor therapy practitioners to adopt the best available evidence for improving psychotherapy outcomes and to champion being able to claim that our field implements the very best available evidence as to what helps improve our clients' outcomes. In some ways, we have. Our ecopsychological underpinnings, presented in Chapters 1 and 3, offer a depth in understanding of well-being that may be missing from other schools of therapy. However, positioning our practice on the mantle of the best-available evidence can help navigate our field toward incorporating aspects of practice designed to improve the therapeutic work we are doing.

Too often knowledge from bordering fields is used to inform the outdoor therapies and many of these studies are cited throughout this book. For example, there is clearly a breadth of evidence suggesting that time spent in the outdoors and connection to nature can generate significant benefits to health and well-being. Unfortunately, however, there is lack of evidence to suggest therapy conducted in outdoor settings will produce better outcomes, as direct comparison trials have found equivalent quantitative outcomes for therapy conducted in both settings (Dobud & Harper, 2018). Embracing the available evidence and incorporating it into practice is not only central to many of our professional standards of practice, but also can be used to help therapists develop plans to improve outcomes for clients, something most therapists would like to do (Miller et al., 2015). We believe that for the outdoor therapies to gain further recognition as a bona-fide mode of psychotherapy, embracing the current evidence and building the best-available knowledge base is required. This means exploring the relationship of the therapeutic alliance to outcomes, dose-effect, therapist effects, dropout rates, and deterioration.

It is important in concluding this section that we are not arguing for one way of knowing, though we acknowledge the potential positivist slant to this discussion; funny given at this stage we are two qualitative scholars early in our academic careers calling for the implementation of the best available evidence for improving outcomes. The popularity of postmodernism stances has given rise to models of therapy like solution-focused brief therapy and narrative therapy, both of which have influenced the outdoor therapies (Knowles, 2013; Natynczuk, 2016). That said, adopting a postmodern approach does not inform practitioners to wholly discount scientific pursuits in psychotherapy, but to embrace the many ways of knowing which ground the evidence we use to support our practice.

Given the promise of outcome monitoring and the effects of approaches like Feedback-Informed Treatment in improving outcomes over time (Miller et al., 2015), we see this as a good example of what outdoor therapy practitioners can do to embrace the evidence. Along with embracing the available evidence, we felt a brief revisiting of ethics was timely for concluding this book.

Ethical Considerations

Many of the chapters in this book had space for some discussion of ethics. For example, Heather White and Kay Scott in Chapter 9 developed a discussion of not only ethical views for clients but also the animals practitioners may invite into therapy. Ethical considerations for taking therapy outdoors have been discussed previously in the literature and suggest further exploration is needed (Harper, Rose et al., 2019; Hooley, 2016). In Chapter 14, Denise Mitten brought forward important considerations about the dated language used in our field, and raised concerns about the concepts of comfort zone, challenge by choice, and what she described as paternal models of service delivery. Mitten also challenged the field to adopt diverse perspectives and move past the Euro-centric and patriarchal dominant paradigms that have guided many outdoor therapies for too long.

We build on Mitten's presentation of ethical considerations in effort to broaden this dialog. We encourage that outdoor therapists consider adopting increased standards for oversight and focus on the physical and psychological safety of the client, and specialized training and education. Some practices described in this book take place in remote areas, far from where traditional talk therapy sessions generally take place. Some of this work takes place in more populated areas, such as surfing with young clients on a populated beach or walking through a park in an urban environment. In each setting, ethical practice may look different than office-based therapies.

While all individual therapy tends to take place behind a closed door, outdoor therapies require further considerations due to issues of supervision and oversight. In these settings, practitioners may not be held to the same ethical standards as those practicing in clinics in urban environments. This has certainly been the case for residential treatment and wilderness therapy in the United States where a lack of regulation and oversight has resulted in young client deaths and practices which may be at odds with most therapeutic professional associations (Becker, 2010). An example of how to offer increased oversight to improve the safety of the client comes from the U.S. State of Utah which has crafted strong safety regulations for therapeutic programs offered in wilderness areas. This set of rules provides basic safety through a list of required expedition planning, mandated personal equipment, protocols for medical care, and daily logs. Staff are required to hold minimum requirements for education, experience, age (18 at the youngest), emergency response training, and other criteria for employees at all levels of the organizations, volunteers included. Young clients also require prior medical examinations and guaranteed access to standards of nutrition and hydration while in the outdoor youth program. These thorough and extensive laws regulating programs in Utah could be utilized as an example for those who provide outdoor therapies in currently unregulated areas.

Of course, not all outdoor therapy programs take place in remote and isolated locations. The contributing authors throughout this book provided descriptions of outdoor therapies offered in outdoor locations in or near populated centers. The approaches can experience equally unique ethical challenges, such as how to protect client confidentiality, supervisory oversight and support, and protecting the safety of the client and practitioner. In these locations it is likely that the delivery of an outdoor therapy may be observed by others. Client confidentiality is a key ethical concern here. The therapist must recognize that just their presence with a client in settings where they can be observed by the community may violate client confidentiality, especially in smaller populations where clients may know many members of their community. Therapists, in this case, should take special care to find locations where they can provide outdoor therapy services with a level of privacy and discuss often with clients this possibility and plan accordingly how to deal with it.

There are times in therapy where a therapist may need support from their supervisory team, such as a client crisis or other issue that arises during an outdoor therapy session. This could provide challenges when offering therapy outdoors away from the support of the team and supervisors. Practitioners and supervisors should establish protocols for supervisor consultation and crisis support while offering outdoor therapy services.

Education and training is another area where outdoor therapies can strive for improved ethical standards. Unethical practice could occur when programs employ those without proper education and training to provide effective outdoor therapy services. Terms such as adventure therapist, nature-based therapist, or wilderness therapist are often not protected terms that require practitioners hold professional degrees. However, the necessary skills for outdoor therapy often necessitate that practitioners have received formal education in both therapeutic skills and outdoor safety skills and these skills are rarely offered in the same university education program. Also, those offering outdoor therapeutic services come from a wide array of professional backgrounds that include medicine, many helping professions, education, and other social services. Training levels and requirements vary widely across programs. One program may use 'therapeutic' guides that are recent-high school graduates with adventure-based certifications while others may require those with graduate degrees and extensive psychotherapeutic training.

The field of outdoor therapies is likely too large for overarching recommendations for training to be implemented across the board. What we recommend is that each outdoor therapy organization consult with local professional boards and associations to adopt their own standards of education that include both professional therapeutic skills as well as technical outdoor skills suitable for the activities they offer. These standards should reflect those recommended by local laws as well as professional boards.

Conclusion

Any professional group not keeping pace with advancements of research and technology is likely destined for extinction. While sections of this book have discussed the negative consequences of urbanization and technification, as advocates of taking therapy outdoors, we also acknowledge the need to continuing adapting; holding ourselves and our peers accountable to changing theories and practice, and moving this exciting field into the future in a professional and ethical manner.

References

Annerstedt, M. & Währborg, P. (2011). Nature-assisted therapy: Systematic review of controlled and observational studies. *Scandinavian Journal of Public Health*, 39(4), 371–388.

Becker, S. P. (2010). Wilderness therapy: Ethical considerations for mental health professionals. *Child and Youth Care Forum*, 39(1), 47–61.

Becker, S. P. & Russell, K. C. (2016). Wilderness therapy. In R. J. R. Levesque (Ed.), *Encyclopedia of adolescence* (2nd ed., pp. 1–10). Cham, Switzerland: Springer International.

Beightol, J., Jevertson, J., Carter, S., Gray, S., & Gass, M. (2012). Adventure education and resilience enhancement. *Journal of Experiential Education, 35*, 307–325.

Bell, E. (2015). Young persons in research: A call for engagement of youth in mental health research. *The American Journal of Ethics in Research, 15*, 28–30.

Bettmann, J. E., Russell, K. C., & Parry, K. J. (2013). How substance abuse recovery skills, readiness to change and symptom reduction impact change processes in wilderness therapy participants. *Journal of Child and Family Studies, 22*(8), 1039–1050.

Bettmann, J. E., Gillis, H. L., Speelman, E. A., Parry, K. J., & Case, J. M. (2016). A meta-analysis of wilderness therapy outcomes for private pay clients. *Journal of Child and Family Studies, 25*, 2659–2673.

Bowen, D. J. & Neill, J. T. (2013). A meta-analysis of adventure therapy outcomes and moderators. *The Open Psychology Journal, 6*, 28–53.

Burke, N. J., Hellman, J. L., Scott, B. G., Weems, C. F., & Carrion, V. G. (2011). The impact of adverse childhood experiences on an urban pediatric population. *Child Abuse & Neglect, 35*, 408–413.

Caldwell, B. E. (2015). *Saving psychotherapy: How therapists can bring the talking cure back from the brink.* Los Angeles, CA: Ben Caldwell Labs.

Carter, S. L., Straits, J. E., & Hall, M. (2007). *Project venture: Evaluation of a positive, culture-based approach to substance abuse prevention with American Indian youth.* Technical Report. Gallup, NM: The National Indian Youth Leadership Project.

Chow, D. L., Miller, S. D., Seidel, J. A., Kane, R. T., Thornton, J. A., & Andrews, W. P. (2015). The role of deliberate practice in the development of highly effective psychotherapists. *Psychotherapy, 52*, 337–345.

Dobud, W. (2017). Towards an evidence-informed adventure therapy: Implementing feedback-informed treatment in the field. *Journal of Evidence-Informed Social Work, 14*, 172–182.

Dobud, W. & Harper, N. J. (2018). Of dodo birds and common factors: A scoping review of direct comparison trials in adventure therapy. *Complementary Therapies in Clinical Practice, 31*, 16–24.

Dobud, W. W. (2020). *Narratives of the co-adventurers: The collaborative explorations of adolescent experiences in adventure therapy* (Unpublished doctoral dissertation). Charles Sturt University, Wagga Wagga, Australia.

Dobud, W. W., Cavanaugh, D. L., & Harper, N. J. (2020). Adventure therapy and routine outcome monitoring of treatment: The time is now. *Journal of Experiential Education.* Advance online publication. doi:10.1177/1053825920911958

Dube, S. R., Anda, R. F., Felitti, V. J., Edwards, V. J., & Croft, J. B. (2002). Adverse childhood experiences and personal alcohol abuse as an adult. *Addictive Behaviors, 27*, 713–725.

Goldberg, S. B., Rousmaniere, T., Miller, S. D., Whipple, J., Nielsen, S. L., Hoyt, W. T., & Wampold, B. E. (2016). Do psychotherapists improve with time and experience? A longitudinal analysis of outcomes in a clinical setting. *Journal of Counseling Psychology, 63*, 1–11.

Gass, M. A., Gillis, H. L., & Russell, K. C. *Adventure therapy: Theory, Research, and Practice.* Routledge.

Gillis, H. L., Speelman, E., Linville, N., Bailey, E., Kalle, A., Oglesbee, N., ... & Jensen, J. (2016). Meta-analysis of treatment outcomes measured by the Y-OQ and Y-OQ-SR comparing wilderness and non-wilderness treatment programs. *Child & Youth Care Forum, 45*(6), 851–863.

Hannan, C., Lambert, M. J., Harmon, C., Nielsen, S. L., Smart, D. W., Shimokawa, K., & Sutton, S. W. (2005). A lab test and algorithms for identifying clients at risk for treatment failure. *Journal of Clinical Psychology, 61*(2), 155–163.

Harper, N. J. (2017). Wilderness therapy, therapeutic camping and adventure education in child and youth care literature: A scoping review. *Children and Youth Services Review, 83,* 68–79.

Harper, N. J., Mott, A. J., & Obee, P. (2019). Client perspectives on wilderness therapy as a component of adolescent residential treatment for problematic substance use and mental health issues. *Children and Youth Services Review, 105,* 104450.

Harper, N. J., Rose, K., & Segal, D. (2019). *Nature-based therapy: A practitioner's guide to working outdoors with children, youth, and families.* Gabriola Island, Canada: New Society Publishers.

Hawton, K., Saunders, K. E., & O'Connor, R. C. (2012). Self-harm and suicide in adolescents. *The Lancet, 379,* 2373–2382.

Hooley, I. (2016). Ethical considerations for psychotherapy in natural settings. *Ecopsychology, 8*(4), 215–221.

Howard, K. I., Moras, K., Brill, P. L., Martinovich, Z., & Lutz, W. (1996). Evaluation of psychotherapy: Efficacy, effectiveness, and patient progress. *American Psychologist, 51*(10), 1059–1063.

International Surf Therapy Organization. (2019). International surf therapy organization: Go far together. Retrieved June 10, 2019 from https://intlsurftherapy.org

Knowles, B. (2013). Journeys in the bush. *International Journal of Narrative Therapy & Community Work, 3,* 39–48.

Kutcher, S., Bagnell, A., & Wei, Y. (2015). Mental health literacy in secondary schools: A Canadian approach. *Child and Adolescent Psychiatric Clinics of North America, 24,* 233–244.

Lambert, M. J., Whipple, J. L., Smart, D. W., Vermeersch, D. A., Nielsen, S. L., & Hawkins, E. J. (2001). The effects of providing therapists with feedback on patient progress during psychotherapy: Are outcomes enhanced? *Psychotherapy Research, 11,* 49–259.

Lan, P., Sveen, R., & Davidson, J. (2004). A Project Hahn empirical replication study. *Journal of Outdoor and Environmental Education, 8,* 37–43.

Masten, A. S. (2014) *Ordinary magic: Resilience in development.* New York, NY: Guilford Press.

Meichenbaum, D. & Lilienfeld, S. O. (2018). How to spot hype in the field of psychotherapy: A 19-item checklist. *Professional Psychology: Research and Practice, 49,* 22–30.

Merikangas, K. R. & McClair, V. L. (2012). Epidemiology of substance use disorders. *Human Genetics, 131,* 779–789.

Michalewicz-Kragh, B. (2019) *Evaluation of outcomes following surf therapy.* Retrieved 19 June, 2019 from https://clinicaltrials.gov/ct2/show/NCT02857751

Miller, S. D., Hubble, M. A., Chow, D. L., & Seidel, J. A. (2013). The outcome of psychotherapy: Yesterday, today, and tomorrow. *Psychotherapy, 50*(1), 88–97.

Miller, S. D., Hubble, M. A., Chow, D., & Seidel, J. (2015). Beyond measures and monitoring: Realizing the potential of feedback-informed treatment. *Psychotherapy, 52*(4), 449–457.

Miller, S. D. & Schuckard, E. (2014). Psychometrics of the ORS and SRS: Results from the RCT's and meta-analyses of routine outcome monitoring & feedback. The available evidence [Slides]. Retrieved June 12, 2020 from http://www.slideshare.net/scottdmiller/measures-and-feedback-miller-schuckard-2014

Modecki, K. L., Minchin, J., Harbaugh, A. G., Guerra, N. G., & Runions, K. C. (2014). Bullying prevalence across contexts: A meta-analysis measuring cyber and traditional bullying. *Journal of Adolescent Health, 55*, 602–611.

Monnat, S. M. & Chandler, R. F. (2015). Long-term physical health consequences of adverse childhood experiences. *The Sociological Quarterly, 56*, 723–752.

National Association of Social Workers. (2017). Code of ethics. Retrieved 10 August, 2019 from https://www.socialworkers.org/About/Ethics/Code-of-Ethics/Code-of-Ethics-English

Natynczuk, S. (2016). Solution-focused practice as a useful addition to the concept of adventure therapy. *InterAction, 6*(1), 23–36.

Psychotherapy and Counselling Federation of Australia [PACFA]. (2013). *Evidence-informed practice statement.* Retrieved August 14, 2019 from https://www.pacfa.org.au/research/evidence-based-practice-statement/

Riebschleger, J. L., Costello, S., Cavanaugh, D. L., & Grové, C. (2019). Mental health literacy of youth that have a family member with a mental illness: Outcomes from a new program and scale. *Frontiers of Psychiatry, 10*, 1–10.

Riebschleger, J. L., Grové, S., Costello, S., & Cavanaugh, D. L. (2018). Mental health literacy for children with a parent with a mental illness. *Journal of Parent and Family Mental Health, 3*, 1–3.

Ritchie, S. D., Wabano, M. J., Russell, K., Enosse, L., & Young, N. L. (2014). Promoting resilience and wellbeing through an outdoor intervention designed for Aboriginal adolescents. *Rural Remote Health, 14*, 2523.

Schilling, E. A., Aseltine, R. H., & Gore, S. (2007). Adverse childhood experiences and mental health in young adults: A longitudinal survey. *BMC Public Health, 7*, 30.

Scull, J. (2008). Ecopsychology: Where does it fit in psychology in 2009? *The Trumpeter, 24*, 68–85.

Selhub, E. M. & Logan, A. C. (2012). *Your brain on nature: The science of nature's influence on your health, happiness and vitality.* Hoboken, NJ: John Wiley & Sons.

Smith, M. L. & Glass, G. V. (1977). Meta-analysis of psychotherapy outcome studies. *American Psychologist, 32*, 752–760.

Steel, Z., Marnane, C., Iranpour, C., Chey, T., Jackson, J. W., Patel, V., & Silove, D. (2014). The global prevalence of common mental disorders: A systematic review and meta-analysis 1980–2013. *International Journal of Epidemiology, 43*, 476–493.

Wampold, B. E. & Imel, Z. E. (2015). *The great psychotherapy debate: The evidence for what makes psychotherapy work* (2nd ed.). New York, NY: Routledge.

Williams, F. (2017). *The nature fix: Why nature makes us happier, healthier, and more creative.* W. W. Norton & Company.

Index